Miracle of Body Wisdom

How to break through anxiety and reclaim your mind, body and heart.

Joseph Lauricella

Wolf Spirit Publishing—Camillus, NY
ISBN: 979-8-9882467-0-1
eBook ISBN: 979-8-9882467-1-8
Library of Congress Control Number: 2023909962
Title: *Miracle of Body Wisdom*
Author: Joseph Lauricella
Digital distribution | 2023
Paperback | 2023

Illustrations by Junior's Digital Design
Cover Design by Ashley Bilz

*Note: The contents of this book are not meant to diagnose, prescribe, or treat any condition, ailment or illness, mentally, physically or otherwise. The recommendations, tips, instructions, and exercises in this book are in no way intended to be a substitute for medical treatment or a doctor's care. It is recommended that you consult with your physician in all matters of health and especially prior to any exercise, breathwork, movement or nutritional/dietary recommendations found here within. The author, nor the publisher is responsible or liable for any damage, injury, illness, or accident, directly or indirectly, from following the information in this book.

Dedication

I dedicate this book to you, the reader. May the pages ahead help clear the path to peace, love and understanding.

Acknowledgements

I am grateful for my first teachers, my parents for lighting the way straight from the heart and whose love remains present in my life today. To all the teachers who have graced me with their example, knowledge, wisdom and insights throughout my own healing journey. Among them: Chris Melco, who shared his medicine ways when I was a young man questioning my purpose. Servando, who first introduced me to the Inipi Ceremony (sweat lodge) and provided a sanctuary for so many people to come and pray in the hills of Pecos, NM. Dr. Scott Thomas, a Lakota sun dancer who became a friend and mentor. To the late Michael Hopp who was my first Yoga teacher. His influence and inspiration never wanes even to this day. Michael Smith, my first Ashtanga teacher who stressed the importance of pranayama. Reverend Gregory Wiest who taught me the skillful art of writing and then "editing the shit out of it" to share my gifts. A ton of gratitude to all my proofreaders, especially Shirley "Girly" Krohn whose love and support has always felt like family. Laurie Gaetano who swooped in with her eagle eyes and honest feedback. Juli Kimbal who was instrumental in helping with the outline of the book. Ashley Bilz who created the beautiful cover design in record time. A deep bow to all the teachers and sages who have dedicated their lives to the transmission of Yoga in the Great Tradition: Tirumalai Krishnamacharya, TKV Desikachar, J. and UG Krishnamurti and especially to my teacher and friend Mark Whitwell, whose capacity to love and teach is unparalleled. Who wholeheartedly believes that Your Yoga is the hope for our humanity. I am profoundly thankful for your tireless transmission and education of real Yoga to all people worldwide. I am deeply grateful to every single person whom I've had the honor and privilege to work with and teach over the last 25 years in Yoga classes, workshops, retreats or bodywork sessions.

Contents

Introduction

You are the power of the universe! A living, breathing miracle with an extraordinary amount of intrinsic intelligence housed in your body. This is not hyperbole, nor am I interested in reminding you of this fact like good trivia. It's rather an invitation for you to trust your own body's wisdom. The same wisdom that brought you into this world and continues to move through you every second of every day. An invitation for you to feel and accept this truth in every cell of your being.

When you were conceived, a massive amount of information was exchanged that built every aspect of your body, allowing you to see, feel, hear, taste, touch and experience the world. In utero, you were built from the inside, out. Once you were born, you began learning from the outside, in. We all began this journey with little control over our well-being. Shit happened to us, and we experienced things that, maybe, we wish we hadn't. As we grew up, we developed internal mechanisms to navigate and cope with the rough patches while also being shaped by our external circumstances. From the microcosm of our family unit to the macrocosm of the rest of the world. Everyone has a story of how they got to where they perceive themselves to be.

Have you ever wondered why some people have all the money they could ever want, yet they're unhappy, while others who have next to nothing are always smiling? Many spiritual teachers say that it's simply a choice that you make over and over in the present moment. It's the present moment that is so elusive, otherwise we would be able to quickly think our way out of anxiety, grief, depression and an overactive mind. Our body is our real biography, and it often tells a different story than the one we maintain. This discrepancy can create an internal dialogue that is difficult to turn off or understand.

I have experienced the pitfalls of dealing with my own mental turmoil that nearly cost me my life. I have also worked with thousands of people who want nothing more than to quiet the busy voice in their head and accept their body regardless of its condition. Quieting the mind and trusting the body's wisdom is the key that unlocks the doors of perception. When we manually link the brain to the body it begins a purifying process as natural as a bird cleaning and maintaining its feathers, or a dog stretching after a deep sleep. With pure intention, worry, fear, attachment, unawareness, and the constant search to make life perfect, begins to drop away.

The wisdom of the body already knows how to clean up and clear out, given the chance. When we make the conditions right, the mind quiets down and we align to the spirit-self in the present moment the way we did as an infant. A time before you were programed by trauma and defense mechanisms. Before the culture conditioned you to be separate from your heart and the miracle that makes it beat.

This book is about calling you home to reunite you to the purity of your spirit, and the truth of your body no matter how old you are, or what shape you're in. It's to guide you back to the innocence and natural state from which you came. A place free of worry and too many thoughts. A place where you don't need armor or perfection or any standard whatsoever. When you spend some time in this natural state regularly, I have faith that it will be easier to choose love over fear no matter what happened or has not happened in your life. After all, we don't have to go looking for happiness and peace, it already lives inside of us. We can trust the ancient intelligence that brought us here.

Trust me, I did not always believe this myself. In fact, in the pages ahead I share my story, which was a bitter internal battle until I hit bottom. It took a near death experience and several days in the hospital before I began questioning the lies that I had believed about myself. Then it took me years to understand that I, like you, have been programmed like a computer and some of that programming can be destructive. If we don't update our "system" along life's journey, we get stuck in the old paradigms of the past and develop new worries about the future. If we don't have a consistent practice that unites us with and actualizes our present condition, no matter what that is, we will likely suffer.

Most of us were conditioned to believe that the answers to life are outside of our own body and being. We were indoctrinated into a culture that sends us out on a never-ending search to make ourselves happy. It's even written in the U.S. Declaration of Independence: "…life, liberty and the pursuit of happiness."

Ironically, for many it's the pursuit that makes us miserable. When we let go of the quest to find happiness and peace outside of ourselves and embrace what we already are, suffering ends. The wisdom keepers and realizers like, Buddha, Jesus, and Gandhi lived and carried this message through the ages. It was shared in oral traditions of indigenous cultures around the world and has been written in various religious texts in one way or another: *Your body is a temple that houses your spirit, and you can't have true happiness without inner peace.*

Peace is already our natural state, but we have been duped into believing we need certain things deemed by our society for us to be happy and peaceful. What we don't think we have or what everyone else has, we go searching for it, and that search often separates us from the truth of what we already are.

In our consumer driven culture, we grow up believing that we need things and achievements to fill a void inside of us. A void that does not actually exist. The nature of a highly competitive society cannot help, but to implant the idea that you are not good enough, you don't have enough and you're not doing enough. From a young age we are filled with expectations of others and spend our lives trying to prove to the world our worthiness. The pandemic brought this to the surface, because it took away all the distractions. Suddenly, people were forced to interact more intimately with their internal voices.

Stress, anxiety and depression are themselves a symptom of these times. They are a lofty expression of self-denial and disassociation from the truth of our own miracle of life. Instead of seeking refuge in our own body, we run from it, bully it, stuff it and judge it. Instead of hearing our stress and anxiety as a voice calling us inward, we view it as something we need to get rid of. Instead of validating this voice as part of us, we try to shut it up and shut it out. Instead of embracing the scared, worried child inside of us that does not feel safe, we run from them, or worse, turn our backs on him or her. Too often, we ignore or try to cover up these deeper parts of ourselves.

What if we just listened? Listened to the voice of fear and worry? What if we learned how to make peace with these scared parts of ourselves? What if we embraced all parts of ourselves with unconditional love? What if we called bullshit on the lies and stories that have been zapping our energy? What if we re-engineered our mind to allow our body to be a safe space?

Every solid, stable relationship is built on trust and good communication.

The truth is: there's an ancient timeless wisdom coursing through us. We are literally the power of the universe itself. We have instant access to this great power and it's not out there in the world to be searched for, it's inside of our own body. Our body must become our sanctuary if we want to transform stress, anxiety, and overthinking into peace, empowerment and love.

My mission is to help you cultivate your inner sanctuary with an intimate, daily practice. A practice that reminds you of the vast intelligence that you are. A practice that conveys this without the idea that you have to attain something better or get to someplace special. Instead, I am called here to help you accept and shape your miracle of life. Learning to love yourself in this unique way, unconditionally, is the single most important thing any one of us can do for our self, our family, and our planet.

Chapter 1
You Are A Miracle

I am once again sitting at a picnic table surrounded by trees in the middle of the Adirondack Mountains. It's autumn. The leaves parachute down on their final descent to the ground. The bright red colors in the trees are the ones you see on postcards and canvases. The peculiar smell of decay lingers in the cool air as winter approaches. The geese are resting in the pond on their way south to warmer states. We're heading in the same direction following the warmth of the sun. I'm still on the road.

When the Covid pandemic hit, I was living in Chicago, teaching big Yoga classes and enjoying my life. Within two weeks I lost my job, my apartment, and my relationship. Aside from illness or poor health, I was hit with the three biggest causes of stress and anxiety all at once. So, I did what anyone in their right mind would do. I bought an old school bus, converted it into a rolling Yoga studio and hit the road. I taught Yoga down the eastern seaboard all the way to south Florida. I also started offering Yoga/Meditation Retreats again. The retreats provide a space for people to come home, find refuge in their own body, and once again align the mind to the heart.

There is a spiritual void and mental health crisis in the United States and much of the world today. The increasing numbers of anxiety, depression, suicide, tribalism, gun violence, and addiction are all symptoms of humanity's disassociation from our own reality.

Reality is what is actually occurring in space and time, which is your body. Spirituality is the realization that we are reality. Our body is literally the purest form of reality, and it runs on electricity in the form of nerve impulses and intelligence. A spiritual practice then, is to acknowledge and honor our body that contains and interacts with the energy of the universe. This is a whole body and breath experience. In fact, if we hold our attention on the body and breath interplay for a long enough period of time, the mind systematically begins releasing patterns of obstruction and worry, stored trauma and tension. This provides enough space for new insight to move in and our burdens to move out. Though it can be challenging to have the discipline to actually do a daily practice while entangled with everything that's happening in your life, it's also the best time.

The spiritual retreats that I offer, give people an opportunity to see things with fresh eyes. Clear out the clutter of the mind and experience the body in a profoundly nurturing and restful way. When we create some literal distance between our regular daily life of a: home, job, chores, finance, relationship, and kids with consecutive days dedicated to the simplicity of self-care and rest, a shift naturally occurs. This shift allows you a new perspective on everything that has happened in your life as well as what you want to bring into it. Most people leave the retreat not only feeling lighter, grounded in their body, and aligned, but inspired to do a daily practice that clears the mind, lifts your spirits and re-instates the truth.

Here's the truth: You began life as two cells. Two tiny, microscopic cells. One from each parent. Those two cells all by themselves multiplied to give you a beating heart, brain, central nervous system and so on. You have grown to over 30 trillion cells all specialized to harness and allow electricity to flow through you to give you life. This life takes form within and around your body. It is extreme intelligence. It is and you are literally source energy. You came from nothing, a mystery of sorts.

In fact, you are the definition of a miracle! The chance of you being alive is one in four hundred quadrillion. The probability of you having a body and breathing air as a human being is as close to zero as it can be. Yet, you are here. Please understand the significance of this. You are an extraordinary embodiment. You have a vast intelligence system. You are an organism like no other living thing on the planet. You are a divine integration of source materials in the most deliberate sophisticated formula known to exist. You are source energy, and you are connected to everything in the universe. You are part of a dynamic web that weaves through all things. You literally have a far better chance of winning Powerball on any given day than being born at the exact time that you were.

Do you live your life feeling as if you won the lottery every day? Most people don't. We have all sorts of reasons why this doesn't feel true, nevertheless, it is. Numbers don't lie and the chance of you being here at all, let alone reading these words is not some random roll of the dice.

When you were conceived, source perfectly aligned with the physical manifestation of you and it's undeniable, because you are actually here. You materialized out of nothing. You are not a mistake even if your parents did not plan on having you. No matter what the circumstances were when you were conceived you were meant to be here. The action you take from this point forward will make a difference in your life, your family's life and the very planet on which you live. If you decide to continue reading and implement the practices in this book, a positive shift will undoubtedly occur in your life.

A shift in your perspective, perception and your ability to see more clearly. An upgrade in the way you communicate with yourself, express yourself, and honor your gift of life. A better understanding and connection to your own body's structure and function. You will come to realize that your past does not define you and only exists as a story. Perhaps most importantly, you'll come to know, rely on, and seek refuge in your own body. Instead of disassociating from your body's intelligence, you'll learn to embrace it, care for it, and rest deeply in it.

When you take your attention off of trying to get rid of your stress, anxiety, or depression, and place it on your miracle of life, you will return to love. Self-love is the most important love that you can have. Learning to love yourself unconditionally, no matter how old you are, where you came from, what happened, how much money you have, what you look like, or how many followers you have is the single most important thing any one of us can do for our self, our family, and the planet full stop.

When you tune into what you received first in life and make it a daily practice, a re-alignment takes place. This intimacy with self: body, breath and relationship is a healing endeavor. This is Yoga, the ancient technology given to humans by wisdom keepers to participate, assimilate and actualize our current reality. This is the hope for humanity.

Before we dive into the main content, I want to share with you how I got here. It was not by accident, nothing is.

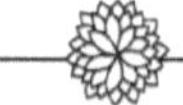

Chapter 2
Best Friends

There are times in our life when it feels like the ground beneath us crumbles, often produced by a traumatic event, accident or illness. Times when a sudden shift occurs and the life we were living is altered forever. Everyone has childhood trauma. The circumstances might be different and certainly some are more severe than others, yet the body's reactions are innate. Our core feelings are the same. We all create defense mechanisms and survival strategies from what happened. We develop automatic responses to cope with the after affects that linger on in our thoughts and body, whether it's a clinical form of PTSD or not.

I'm from a large Italian family, so death was not new to me. I have carried my share of caskets from the time I was a teenager. I had experienced many of my relatives passing, but it wasn't until my best friend, Paul, committed suicide that I began to understand grief and suffering on a deeper level. I was 20 years old. His sudden death strangely gave me my purpose, but I didn't know that then.

Paul's father and mine grew up together. Paul was actually a few years older than me. He was originally closest to my oldest brother. Paul suffered from what millions of people suffer from today: acute anxiety, obsessive compulsive disorder (OCD), depression, and hopelessness. He was stuck in his head overthinking everything. Despite knowing more and openly discussing mental health in various forums, the numbers of people struggling with mental health today continues to climb.

Paul was in a fight every day. He did his best to be okay in the world, to hold his shit together so to speak. His overactive mind was relentlessly spitting out too many thoughts like a printer kicking out the same page over and over. These thoughts led to feelings of despair and inadequacy. On more than one occasion he talked about suicide as a way out of the overwhelming thoughts and feelings that he was unable to control. He was conflicted by his inner world experience and what was actually happening in the outer world. We all tried to help. My family often discussed what we could do to support him, but we just didn't know. My brothers and I often acted like interpreters doing our best to explain the reality of his given situation, which often opposed his inner world thought process. We kept reiterating to him that he was okay despite him not thinking that he was. Being out of touch with reality and disassociated from the truth is not only a symptom of people experiencing anxiety, it's a symptom of our current culture.

Over time, Paul looked to me for emotional support and encouragement. He was in a type of pain that I had no way of understanding at the time, but I tried. To the best of my ability, I tried. As hard as it was to spend so much time with a person who was in so much pain, I was committed. Perhaps stubbornly so. It was the late 80's. Mental health was a new topic and rarely discussed openly the way it is today. I listened to Paul talk through what he was experiencing for hours at a time. I tried to understand his experience, feel what he was feeling. I wanted him to know that he was not alone on the battlefield of his mind fighting an un-winnable war. It was a heavy load to carry as a teenager, but he was my friend and I felt compelled to be there for him.

Although it was not my responsibility, it was clearly my destiny. Life is like that sometimes, isn't it? The reason why things happen may not be revealed for years to come. Our job is to look for and trust that something good will emerge from something seemingly bad. This is faith. Even though we may not always know what to do, something inside of us does. The question is: how do we get ourselves out of the way to trust this voice, this inner knowing, our intuition?

For some reason, I was able to trust this voice then. I know now why I had to go through the pain and suffering in the aftermath. It led me on my own healing journey. My hope is that this book will help you on yours, so that you can move forward in your own life with less resistance and more trust, less angst and more peace.

Paul and I spent many long nights and early mornings driving, talking and listening to music until the sun came up. He confided in me completely up until a few weeks before he took his own life. He would tell me the thoughts he struggled with every day. Self-sabotaging, self-defeating thoughts and most were not even true. He had irrational fears and phobias about germs, about food, about batteries, about vomiting. He didn't work much, but when he did, he'd dose himself with six shots of vodka before making sandwiches at the sub shop. Most people would be drunk, but he functioned normally. He was in and out of treatment and on and off medication. He hated them both. He felt stigmatized. Paul was so intelligent that he often did his own research and diagnosed himself long before Google became a search engine. His psychiatrists often sat across from him scratching their heads about how to help him. He lost hope. This is a characteristic that nearly all suicidal people share. They are unable to see a future for themselves in any way. When you don't have anything to look forward to you begin to look alternatively for a way out of being in constant mental turmoil. He had no purpose. I often helped Paul paint a bright picture of the future, but over time he never made that picture his own. He just never saw a future for himself, because he could not see past his own suffering.

There were times in our interactions that I got frustrated. It seemed like there was nothing I could say or do that made a difference. I became so desperate that I made promises. Promises that would later cause me to feel guilt like being stabbed with a hot serrated edged knife.

One day I finally broke and exclaimed:

"Paul, you can't kill yourself, because you'll be killing me too."

I wanted him to know that the consequence of him committing suicide would be my death as well, as I would take my own life. I meant it. I figured that he'd at least pause before he made an attempt.

I did not know what else to do. I did not have the skills or wisdom to help in any significant way other than to just listen. For a time, I was able to challenge his thoughts, which were mostly lies and give him enough hope to live another day, but he wore me down. Week after week, month after month, a year, another year went by. It became overwhelming and I think he knew. He distanced himself from everyone who loved him. I did not hear from him for a few weeks. He was held up at his parents 'house, which I knew wasn't good. They continued to enable him instead of holding him accountable, but it was too late by then. When I called there, his folks made excuses for him and said that he was not up to talking. I knew this was not a good sign, but I was powerless.

One day when his parents were both gone. Paul was alone with all of his self-defeating thoughts. They took him over. He broke into his father's gun cabinet, took out a shotgun and pulled the trigger. It was a thought that he had rehearsed in his mind far too many times.

A person can only take so much pain and suffering. Paul's mind was out of balance. On one hand he was a genius. He invented, on paper, several electronic components that would eventually make it to the marketplace years later. On the other hand, he had phobias, OCD, and food issues that would stop him in his tracks and keep him isolated from the outside world, from socializing.

His basic needs were constantly interrupted with self-sabotaging thoughts and fear that led to panic attacks. To this day I'm not sure what was at the root of Paul's anxiety, but I do know what was driving it: the belief that he was different than everyone else. It caused him to feel separate or strange and he found evidence to prove it. Whether it was things his friends had said to him over the years or that he was good at manipulating his parents. Instead of finding ways to create boundaries and stand up for himself, he hid. Hiding is a telltale sign that something is off.

For a while, I served as his guide, but he needed, as we all do, something to look forward to. A vision of the future that he could see clearly and adopt as his own. I know it may sound cliche, but happiness is a choice, and it depends on what thoughts we choose to think. Paul rarely just enjoyed life in the moment. He never had that clarity. Without it, it's easy to get buried in the daily grind of too many thoughts and worries that produce confusion, paralysis, and a shut down in the body's channels that allow energy to flow to and from the heart.

My life came to a screeching halt when Paul died. Survivor's guilt took me over. Riddled with anger, grief, and loss, I was crippled. I too lost the ability to see a bright future. So, I took the path of least resistance and used what was available. Drugs and alcohol numbed my pain. They became my new best friend and I self-medicated daily. I'm not proud of it, but it was a part of my process. I should have been in therapy right away, but it was a different era. Tony Soprano from the TV show: *The Sopranos,* had not yet made going to therapy a normal practice, especially for men. I hid my pain from everyone, but especially my parents. Besides, they didn't know how to help me. I was a mess and felt alone. I flirted with death myself many times, as I had promised and every day that I didn't do it, my guilt was amplified. I took chances, walked on the edge of drop offs, sped around corners in my car, drank myself into alcohol poisoning. My friends at the time called me reckless, but it was how I punished myself for not fighting harder. As angry as I was at him, I was even more angry at myself. I hated myself. It was a dark lonely place. I had a nagging voice in my head,' You couldn't save him. You failed. You gave up. You should have done more.'

Over and over. It drove me nuts. So, I grabbed for anything I could get my hands on, a cigarette, a whiskey bottle, a beer, a joint, a drug. I even became addicted to lifting weights. I worked out three times per day, stayed out until the bars closed and worked two jobs. I stayed busy but was driving myself into the ground. I sensed at the time that I was not well, because whenever I stopped moving and doing, all those negative thoughts appeared from behind the veil of my busyness. It sounded like a room full of people talking in my head. Just because you stop moving doesn't mean the brain stops thinking. Not at all. This can perpetuate anxiety and mental disturbances that can translate into our body. You might end up with strange physical urges, sensations or behaviors. Physical manifestations of anxiety could be going to the bathroom often or at certain times whether or not you really have to go. Or feeling strange pains or disturbances in the body that have no diagnosis. Not knowing how we feel or what is happening inside of us is a form of stress in the system. Staying constantly busy and not knowing how to relax can be a defense mechanism. Personally, I had overwhelming thoughts that kept me on the move.

Do you notice any nagging voices in your head? Are they loving and positive or sabotaging? Is your brain constantly talking talking talking? Going over and over something that occurred in the past or worried about the future? Some of these voices are so deep, that we don't even know they're there. This is how you can get stuck in a time frame unable to move past some episode or traumatic life event. Living in the shock waves of trauma often still locked in the body. This can leave a person feeling unsafe in their own body. If it's unsafe to feel sensations in the body, it's common to dissociate in different ways, which tends to separate the body from the brain.[1] When we slow down and become still, the mind and body naturally begin to align, in other words we feel more, and emotions begin to surface. Instead of giving them a way out, we might do something to stop or stuff them, like overeat or drink in excess. It's easy to misinterpret sensations in our body. We also come up with all sorts of ways to steer or deflect people away from what we're really feeling. We might say or do something that throws them off of the truth to avoid feeling exposed. Sometimes we stop our feelings, because we think there's something wrong with us, when it may very well be the opposite. The body has a natural desire to move those emotions through. No feelings are really negative, they just are, and our job is to let them move through us without attaching to them, but we are not taught how to do this. In fact, as we become adults, we are generally conditioned to do the opposite. Hold it together. Be strong. Hold it in. Be tough. Be a rock. Don't cry. Don't get angry. Don't lose face.

---

[1] Bessel Van Der Kolk,M.D.,2014 The Body Keeps The Score, 268-269

In order to do so, we begin a pattern of distraction and disassociation. This is when our brain and body separate. Our body has no way of being in the past or future, yet our mind does. This causes separation and therefore suffering on some level whether we're aware of it or not. The energy of those emotions have a lifecycle. Energy doesn't just disappear or dissolve, it naturally wants to flow. Sometimes these feelings are just too painful, instead of allowing them to move all the way through us, the energy can get lodged in the body. When we don't fully process through all the emotions and aftermath of major shifts, traumas, or hardships in life, a negative inner dialogue can easily be created out of it, because energy must go somewhere. Those thoughts become stories and those stories play like a broken record over and over again keeping the emotion stuck in the body. When we disassociate from the body where these emotions reside we run the risk of both mental and physical health issues or dis-ease. We can even become addicted to negative thought patterns, so we don't have to deal with the pain underneath, despite it contributing negatively to our mental health. We worry about being okay in the future when our past injuries get triggered in the present. We have anxiety and depression, because we have not made peace with our past and or constantly worry about the uncertain future. The present moment is where the magic is, but it can seem elusive unless we take right action and have a safe place to express ourselves.

Chapter 3
The Matter of Mind

Months after Paul died. My folks were away on vacation. I had been at a summer party the night before where I had consumed enough drugs and alcohol to be rendered inebriated. I passed out in a bedroom upstairs. The next morning, I woke up with a golf ball sized lump on the front of my neck. As the day progressed, I developed a fever and chills. The next day I took myself to the doctor. He prescribed me some antibiotics. I went home to rest. Five hours later my parents found me curled up on the living room floor in acute abdominal pain. They rushed me to the hospital where I spent the next ten days.

I was unable to eat, had a fever, and could barely move. The doctors ran tests and more tests. My blood was drawn three times per day every day for seven days. My forearms and hands were bruised from needles and IV's. The skin on the palms of my hands peeled off. I was shot in the butt with demurral, a heavy pain killer, on demand. They struggled to find a diagnosis. There were often a team of doctors standing at the foot of my bed. Their conversation sounded like a *Peanuts* episode. Eventually they said I had a reaction to the one antibiotic pill I took combined with complications from mononucleosis, which I never tested positive for. I never believed them. I did not eat for eight days. I thought I was going to die. The voice of guilt, shame, sadness, and anger was winning the war inside of me. My negative, relentless self-talk literally made me sick.

Ten days was a long time to be with myself, my inner world, especially without food. It was a long time to sift through everything that had happened in my life up to that point. It was in essence, a life review, which is often how people explain their experience at Vipassana, an in-depth ten-day meditation retreat. By the time I returned home from the hospital, I was 20 pounds lighter. I was not a big person to begin with. I was weak, frail and different.

My body may have shrunk, but my consciousness had expanded. I began to see and understand the relationship between my inner world and outer world reality. That my thoughts produced feelings and those feelings drove my actions.

As I lie in that hospital bed some of those thoughts and feelings began to surface:

'You don't deserve to live; you could not even save Paul.'

'You're not worthy of love.'

'You're a failure.'

'No one wants to be around you.'

'You're a piece of shit.'

I literally had made myself sick. Thoughts themselves can suppress the immune system, keep you in a victim mode even if the circumstances happened long ago. Other voices rose to the surface as well, but they were few and spoke softer. They came from someplace else. I noticed them either just before I fell asleep with the rise and fall of my chest as I breathed or as I was waking up from sleep.

'Paul knew how much you cared about him.'

'You were a great friend to him.'

'You have nothing to be ashamed about.'

These words came straight from my heart, the nurturing force of life itself. This is the part of us that we need to stay connected with, but I didn't know how. This is the voice that is always in alignment with our purpose, because it comes from the spirit-self. This is the voice we need to listen to have more access to. It's the innate part of us that is all loving. We can often express kind loving words and sentiments to others who are having a hard time in life, yet we struggle to give the same to ourselves. I wanted to know why?

Although, it took years to fully come to terms with my unraveling. I'll never forget the day I came home from the hospital. It was summer. I stepped out of the car and walked into the house for the first time in nearly two weeks, which felt like two years. I remember the shape of the cracks in the driveway. They looked like lightning bolts. The birds were chirping at full volume. A profound sense of gratitude washed over me. I realized in that moment that gratitude and anxiety cannot co-exist at the same time. It was the first time in my life that I had experienced tears of joy. I wanted to live. It was the beginning of living my life on my own terms, rather than how I was programmed or what was expected of me.

We all have programs running in the background of our mind and they act like recordings from our past. They live in our subconscious and in many ways control our lives. They are in the form of stories and lies that we tell ourselves. Some are created on our own, perhaps as defense mechanisms, others were implanted into us by what we heard other people say at particularly vulnerable times in our lives. Things that we've agreed to that may not actually be true. Especially, if they came from people who had power and control over us or those we looked up to in some way like our parents, family members, teachers, coaches, popular kids, etc. Stuff got into us and often remains unnoticed. Some people can live their whole lives without these stories and lies negatively affecting them, others are more sensitive and experience stress, anxiety and depression. Sometimes they're so deep, so much a part of who we think we are, they go undetected. This is where resentment, fear, and self-punishment often originate.

The more I uncovered what I was telling myself, the easier it became to forgive and love myself through it.

Here are some of the lies I believed over the years and their anecdote or truths.

<u>Lies</u>	<u>Truths</u>
'I don't belong anywhere.'	'I belong everywhere.'
'I am not good enough.'	'I am a miracle.'
'No one wants to be with me.'	'I am never alone.'
'No one listens to me.'	'I am intuitive.'
'I don't know what I'm doing.'	'I trust myself completely.'
'I am a failure.'	'I am extreme intelligence.'
'I am not there yet.'	'I am where I need to be.'

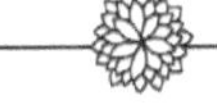

Chapter 4
Coming Home

My most important relationship is with my Source. There is no relationship of greater importance to achieve than the relationship between you, in your physical body, right here and now, and the Soul/Source/God from which you have come. If you tend to that relationship, first and foremost, you will then, and only then, have the stable footing to proceed into other relationships. Your relationship with your own body; your relationship with money; your relationship with your parents, children, grandchildren, the people you work with, your government, your world...will all fall swiftly and easily into alignment once you tend to this fundamental, primary relationship first.

Abraham Hicks

In the years following my hospital stay, I continued to dance with anxiety, depression and negativity. I was able to work but spent my free time hiding from the world alone in my bedroom swimming in residual anger and guilt. I would self-medicate with psychedelics such as marijuana, magic mushrooms, and LSD and read books in search of answers.

I read Carlos Castaneda books like: *Tales of Power* and *A Separate Reality*. I also read: *The Natural Mind* and *Drugs and the Mind*. I dove into Elizabeth Kubler Ross's, *On Death and Dying,* which helped me to better understand the stages of grief.

Most addicts don't start out being dependent on a substance unless their mother was an addict while they were in utero. Most addicts were likely in mental, physical, or emotional pain whether they knew it or not. They either want to feel better or not feel at all. Something happened in their world at some point in their life. Some kind of trauma occurred and they are unable to move forward in their life naturally happy and healthy, they need something to feel good. Therapy can help them put things into context, but talking it out only goes so far, especially if they keep regurgitating the same story over and over. In fact, psychotherapy works ten times better when you're connected to the body.

The combination of reading, writing, walking in the woods and experimenting with mind expansive plant medicines gave way to inspiration. I didn't know it then, but I did the things that I found pleasurable. New ideas would emerge, and I'd leave the cave of my bedroom to set them in motion.

I returned to college to study Sociology and Indigenous American cultures, which led me to the idea to go west. While I fumbled my way through college working a full-time job, I had a vision of buying a van and driving across the country. I didn't really know why. After graduation, I went for it. I had no idea where it would lead me but trusted that it would take me where I needed to go. Living in a van then wasn't nearly as popular as it is today. Even though I read *On The Road* by Jack Kerouac, while I was actually on the road, the world had not yet proliferated it as a lifestyle the way social media depicts it today. Back then, a cross country trip was much more isolating. This was attractive to me as I searched for who I was underneath everything that had been implanted into me. I wanted to shed my conditioning like a skin.

Many of my relatives and friends remarked about how fearless I was, but I really wasn't. I had plenty of fear. Stifling fear in fact. I was afraid that if I did not take a chance and push myself, I would die in my bedroom alone. That thought motivated me enough to force myself outside of my comfort zone. I was also afraid of the unknown. Where would I stay, park, sleep? Who could I trust? Who would I call for help when I'm a thousand miles from home? Yes, I was most certainly afraid.

I hit the road in early Spring of '95, before everyone had a cell phone and a laptop. If I wanted to connect with family or friends, I had to find a pay phone. So yes, it was isolating, but solitude is an important building block in the relationship with self. The first few hours that I drove away from everything that I had ever known was like childbirth. It was as if I passed through some kind of spiritual birth canal. At first, my mind raced. I questioned what the hell I was doing. My shoulders tightened with fear. I felt an enormous amount of pressure in my whole body. For a few hours I sobbed like a baby. It remains today as one of the greatest purging moments of my life. It was as if I shed a skin. Afterwards, something had shifted in me. There was a clearing. I felt a level of peace and clarity I had never experienced.

I spent seven months zigzagging across the Americas mostly alone. I did visit friends living in the west and picked up a few hitchhikers along the way. Some people portrayed me as a lost soul, but I sure didn't feel that way. I felt like an explorer. I ventured into new landscapes and territories on the road and within myself. I felt vital and free. I wrote and published a memoir about my experiences 18 years after I had them in a book titled: *3AM Bull Rider*. In it, I share my experience of asking some of the bigger questions in life.

Who am I? What is my truth underneath my programming? What is my purpose? Some people know the answers to these questions at a young age, but most don't. So, we go find a job that pays the bills, because we want to get started in life. We want to enter the free market and get what everyone else has because we're chasing happiness without really knowing who we are.

I finally landed back at my parents' house looking like Jesus with long hair and a beard. Within six months I enrolled in the New Mexico Academy of Healing Arts School of Massage Therapy. We primarily studied human anatomy and physiology while learning how to make someone feel really good. One of the trademarks of the academy was self-care. This was a powerful combination and set our school apart from others. They insisted that you must care for your own body and mind if you want to help others. *Cur ate ipsum*: "Healer, heal thyself." This is often missing in curriculums that educate people in health care, such as nursing and medical schools. Nursing schools teach students how to care for others, but few if any teach you how to care for yourself, heart and body. In fact, few people are taught how to care for the self on all levels: mentally, physically, emotionally, and spiritually.

The weeks were filled with studying, while weekends were all about prayer and ceremony. I had met a Lakota elder who ran traditional sweat lodge ceremonies on his land in Pecos, NM. This began a massive shift in my life. I experienced new ways of living, seeing, feeling, praying, eating, everything was new and exciting.

Transformation was occurring all around me. In the massage classroom we received therapeutic touch daily. It was like no other place I had ever been. It wasn't just the content of what I learned; it was the environments in which I learned them. It wasn't just about the information from the outside world that entered my mind, it was the wisdom awakened from inside of my own body. There was a deep reverence in the air when you walked down the quiet hallways of the massage school as students released old emotional traumas stored inside their bodies. People were getting to know themselves in a brand-new way as they shed years of baggage, including me. We were all waking up to the realization that our body contains an ancient wisdom and when we set it in motion healing occurs. You have this wisdom inside of your body and when you tap into it and align to your source of power regularly, spontaneous healing occurs.

The healing power of intimate connection is something to behold, because you're working directly with source energy. When the mind finally quiets down and the muscles and organs relax, not only does your body's intelligence initiate repair, release, and detoxification, but a spiritual re-calibration occurs as well. The mind and heart once again align. I say once again, because when you were an infant, they were perfectly aligned. This alignment has a profound effect on the central nervous system, which is especially beneficial for those with mental health concerns. It's not just that you arrive in an extremely relaxed state oblivious to how you got there. It's that you're choosing to nourish your own heart and fully take part in your own life thereby accepting and actualizing reality. By first, taking responsibility for the only things that you can truly own: your heart, body, mind, spirit and emotions.

This level of mindfulness allows you to install a new operating system. One that leaves you feeling uplifted, instead of depressed. Hopeful rather than negative. Grounded and connected to your body instead of anxious and stressed stewing about things in the past or future. The secret to peace and happiness comes directly from first realizing that there's nothing wrong. Initiating a practice of intimate connection will help you let go of the chaos of the external world and go inside. This is how you wake up to, and function in, your current reality no matter what your reality is. Only then can you make the changes that you want.

The first step to waking up and becoming intimate with your own body is to better understand what you have and how it functions. What does it mean when we say the mind/body connection?

When we understand the workings of our extraordinary body and mind, we can take part in and trust it to care for us. The more we participate in the function of the body and breath, the more we contribute and process our life. For most people, it's not our physiological make-up that needs some tweaking, it's our programming/conditioning and perception. Asking the right questions will allow the right answers to surface in time. Instead of asking, how do I get rid of my stress, anxiety, and depression…ask:

Who am I and how do I function? What am I aligned to? How do I practice loving myself unconditionally?

Chapter 5
Our Human Being-ness: What are you?

Knowing what you are made of and how your body generally functions is an important part of taking responsibility for your life. Your body is more than a wonderland, it is an extraordinary organism of profound complexity in its physical, chemical, intuitive, and spiritual integration with the universe. You are made up of over 30 trillion cells. All of which create electricity (voltage) and have the literal ability to transmit energy. You don't have to take an anatomy course to know what you're made out of and generally how your body functions.

Taking responsibility to understand how your body and mind operates is a big deal. I remember taking health class in high school and learning the basics of healthy nutrition and the cardiovascular system, but it all seemed far away from what was taking place inside of me. It wasn't until I thought there was something wrong with me that I began taking more interest in how this incredible organism that we call a body, actually works.

After you were conceived the very first organ cells that assembled to create you, were heart cells. This is important, because as much as the heart is a muscle built to pump blood, it also has specialized cells connected to your emotions. Therefore, your heart is both mechanical and emotional, material and experiential. This will become of great importance on your journey home to the heart, because emotions give us vital information.

What makes your heart, beat? You are electric. Your heart beats, because of an electrical current that rhythmically pulses or sparks over 100,000 times per day. This is the source of your life. In fact, you operate on electricity. From your heartbeat to your ability to think and feel, energy moves throughout your system. You are a vibrational energetic being. You could think of this as tiny sparks taking place inside of your body. When too many sparks accumulate in the brain from overthinking, we experience mental disturbance. A mental overload may trigger a system shut down or malfunction, such as a panic attack. When there's a buildup of energy it can cause your electrical system to short circuit, much like a computer freezes up trying to do too much all at once. Your body acts as if it's in eminent danger, even though it's not.

Along with the construction of your heart came the Central Nervous System (CNS), which by design is an electrical grid system consisting of the brain and spinal cord, which are literally attached to one another. This is a hardwire system for sensory input, information processing, and motor output. If that's too technical, think of your brain as a computer and your spine all the cords hooked up to it giving it power and the ability to connect to the printer and so on. Energy runs to and from the brain through the spinal cord delivering information and sparking or initiating action.

<u>Anatomy of mind, body and spirit.</u>

Have you ever heard the phrase: "we fear what we don't understand?" The unknown keeps us guessing and stuck trying to "figure things out." The opposite of fear is love. Love is a higher form of consciousness than fear. Although this is not an anatomy book per se, I have found that when people have a general understanding of what they're made of and how their own body functions, it gives them relief. Perhaps some of this relief comes from the realization that we're all generally built the same. We have the same anatomy and physiology. This gives people solace that we're never really alone, despite sometimes feeling loss or grief. Compassion for ourselves and others is a natural response to loss, but sometimes anxiety, stress and overthinking perpetuates the idea that everyone else is fine, but you are not. One of the many lies that has found its way into us and we continue to tell ourselves.

The following is an overview of the mind, body and spirit relevant to stress, anxiety and depression. This outlines our basic anatomy and physiology.

Brain vs. mind: The brain is an actual physical structure located inside of our skull bones. The mind is associated with the brain, but not the same thing. The mind is not an actual thing like the brain. The mind involves thought including interpreting, imagining, remembering and the ability to reason. So, when I discuss the mind/body connection, I am referring to the brain's ability in addition to the broad function of the mind relative to consciousness.

<u>Brain: Control Center</u>

Aside from all the involuntary life sustaining operations that the brain does, its primary function is locomotion. This is important as we continue our discussion about mind/body integration and how we will employ moving and being practices.

The brain processes thoughts, behaviors, and perception with cells that function with rapid electrical impulses. It's not surprising that 80% or more of the thoughts you had today were the same thoughts that you had yesterday and the day before that creating a pattern.

Knowing this, it's easy to see how chronic stress and anxiety compounds on itself creating a pattern of fear and worry, this is the pattern that must be interrupted and redirected, repetitively. This is how worry becomes an addiction and when you don't have any real concerns of your own, you might look for something to worry about outside of yourself. Maybe even someone else's problems or struggles. The way we break this unhealthy chain of events is to take back our power, interrupt the cycle and integrate a new way of being with our body and mind.

<u>The main parts of your brain:</u>

<u>Neo-cortex:</u> large part of brain responsible for attention, thought, perception, and episodic memory (everyday events). We can activate the stress response (fight or flight response) just by thinking and worrying about something, because of the capability of the Neo-cortex.

Frontal Lobe: makes up 40% of the brain: emotional expression, cognitive skills, problem solving, memory, language, judgement, sexual behaviors.

Occipital Lobe/ Visual Cortex: allows you to feel in response to emotional stimulus, the Limbic System regulates endocrine (hormone function) and therefore behavior when it comes to survival. Especially fear, anger, hunger, sexual behavior, learning and memory. For this reason chronic stress and anxiety plays a role in high blood pressure among other destructive ailments.

Limbic System includes:
1. Hippocampus -emotional memory
2. Hypothalamus -regulates endocrine & hormone function, especially pituitary and autonomic nervous system, **stress response, and sleep cycles.**
3. Olfactory: sense of smell
4. Thalamus- main relay station, signals sent to and from the spinal cord, seeing, tasting, hearing, touching.
5. **Amygdala – processes fear, anger, pleasure, fear originates here, can be triggered by thoughts, the news, hearing about something scary, it kick starts the stress response.**

The amygdala is an organ that responds as soon as we are in danger. The problem is once these signals are sent, we don't always know the difference between real danger and something we perceive as danger. Our perception is very much based on our programming.

Other Brain Parts:

1. Cingulate gyrus- helps regulate pain and emotion, driving the body's conscious response to unpleasant experiences, avoidance of negative consequences.
2. Cerebellum – coordination, voluntary movements.

From the spinal cord housed in your vertebrae (24 bones + sacrum and tail bones) smaller nerves run throughout the body. These nerves run down the arms and legs into the fingers and toes. They're like wires that carry electricity allowing you to feel and move. This is called the Peripheral Nervous System (PNS).

The Central Nervous System (CNS) has two opposite modes of operation:

(Sympathetic or Automatic) commonly referred to as the Stress Response or the flight, fight, or freeze response.

(Parasympathetic Nervous System) Relaxation Response - rest, digest, peace
*Each mode of the CNS have varying degrees of response.

The Vagus Nerve: works mostly within the parasympathetic Nervous System (rest and digest). It significantly affects heart rate, blood pressure, respiration, immune system, but also influences everything from speech to sensation to digestion. These nerve branches and fibers run from the brain stem down each side of the neck and torso through the diaphragm (breathing muscle) to our organs, especially the stomach. When the Vagus Nerve is conditioned by breathing in certain ways, it can drop us into a Parasympathetic Response creating a calming effect on our mind and body.

The brain and spine are physically attached to one another. They create the mind body connection. When discussing the mind as separate from the body, we're merely speaking about it as an operational phenomenon, because they are physically always connected.

Tony Robins has a saying: "Get in your head and your dead." It's another way of saying that when you overthink or analyze, it's causing you anxiety. It means there's more activity happening in your brain than your mind/body. This occurs when you are trying to figure things out, when your brain is overworking. We can't do all of our processing with the brain alone. Sometimes it's better to feel it out rather than figure it out. We can balance this out in two ways: 1. Move the energy by moving the body. Get the electricity flowing more freely throughout the entire body, rather than having too much electrical stimulation in your brain alone. 2. Breathe and move consciously to calm and move energy. Soothe the amount of stimulation of the electrical activity itself.

<u>Vital Organs and Their Collective Roles</u>
Brain, heart, liver, kidneys, intestines, stomach, lungs, skin, spleen, etc.

1. Detoxification
2. Manufacturing
3. Absorption
4. Elimination
5. Processing

Digestion:

The main role of your digestive system is to process food, absorb nutrients and get rid of waste. Here's the interesting part currently being researched. You not only digest food, you also digest information. There is a direct correlation from mind to gut and gut to mind. Some even say that the stomach is the second brain. Many digestive issues are often caused from stress and your ability to process information and thoughts that create feelings. In fact, when people are in a stress response, the digestive system may partially shut down, causing food and more importantly nutrients not to get absorbed properly. In addition, stress can throw off the healthy gut bacteria that we need to maintain optimal health and immune system function. Even though nutrition plays a significant role in staying healthy in mind and body, the thoughts you think may be more important than the food you eat.

Muscles, bones and connective tissue:

1. The most important muscles in the human body are hands down the heart and diaphragm muscles. The heart is a cardiac muscle. The diaphragm is a skeletal muscle.
2. Skeletal muscles are responsible for locomotion. When muscles contract they get shorter, when they stretch, they elongate. Muscles only pull-on bones, they do not push bones.
3. Muscles, bones, and connective tissue such as tendons, ligaments, and fascia give your body

structure and work together to allow you to move etc.

4. Tendons attach muscles to bones, ligaments attach bone to bone in joints, fascia is the web that weaves through the entire body wrapping around all muscles and organs. Fascia holds us together.
5. Muscles have a direct blood supply. Tendons, ligaments and fascia do not.
6. There are over 640 muscles in the human body. We literally have trillions of nerves that are like wires that run throughout the entire body, all the way to the tips of your fingers and toes.

<u>Your body is a filtration system.</u>

1. Like your vacuum cleaner or furnace has a filter that you change. The filter catches debris. Cleaning out your filters is a key to health.
2. Think about everything that has gone into you from the time you were a child. From information to material, from negative thoughts to toxins, from judgements to chemicals, from I love you to I hate you.
3. From the seen world of material and substances to the unseen world of thoughts and emotions etc.

We all have stories inside of us, some still have emotion tied to them, some don't. Many of the things that have happened in our lives may still be stored in the body in some way. The body in this way is a biography of our lives. The accumulation of what happened leaves behind elements of emotion. We all have some sort of childhood trauma. We have all developed methods to survive those traumas.

Joseph Campbell, Carl Jung, and most recently Bessel van der Kolk have talked about our conditioning and how the body keeps a record of the things that happen to us. Stored or stuck emotions often play a role in our lives. They linger in the background and affect many of our decisions, reactions, and relationships.

Through the years, I have had thousands of bodywork or massage therapy sessions that have triggered a client to have an emotional response through touch. In my experience, this happens when the client has relaxed deeply enough that they're in a heightened state of feeling and allowing. It's when all the defense mechanisms drop away. Feeling is a key to healing. The irony of this statement is that the more you try to feel, the more you may be in your thinking rather than feeling. The body knows how to take care of itself, but this rarely happens in a state of stress or anxiety, it happens in a state of deep relaxation.

Anatomy of the Spirit

What is the spirit? Christians tend to differentiate the spirit from the soul, maintaining that one's spirit is for God and the soul is for the individual. In Hinduism and Buddhism, there's less separation, yet consideration of past life experience, as in some part of us has been here before. For our purposes, it really doesn't matter what you believe. We're talking about energy, source, intelligence, knowledge or spirit taking form and giving us life inside of this body the way it exists right now. I think we can all agree that we have life because we are breathing. Without the breath, there's no life. The word "spirit" comes from the Latin root word: spiritus, meaning: to breathe. Breathing is a spiritual experience and breathing consciously a spiritual practice.

While we all know the importance of mental and physical health, what about spiritual health? We often associate spirituality with religion, but you don't necessarily have to participate or belong to any religion to care for your spirit.

Personally, I grew up Roman Catholic and went to church every week. I knew nothing else for the first 15 years of my life. Eventually, we learn that other belief systems exist. Although, I loved the rituals within the mass, I didn't feel a deep personal connection to the stories and beliefs. I have grown to appreciate the devotional aspect of believing in a higher power. And yes, I love Jesus. I love Buddha too. How could I not have a personal relationship with Jesus? A painting of him or at least what we believe he looked like has been hanging on my parent's bedroom wall since I was born.

However, it wasn't until I was introduced to Lakota Spirituality and later Yoga that I felt something stir inside of me. Perhaps, because my body, mind and breath got involved in ceremony and ritual. I have come to understand that no matter what you believe, we all have an opportunity to connect with our spirit through the very container that holds it, our body and that which keeps it functioning, the breath. This body and breath are in relation to everything else in our lives. We can participate in this movement or flow of life. When we combine conscious controlled breathing with conscious controlled movement, we unite everything that we are: physical, mental, spiritual and emotional.

Spirit:

1. The part of us that is always always loving and supportive.
2. Integrated with breath or to breathe (spiritus).
3. Connection to source: God, creator, divinity, the great mystery or universal energy.
4. Life giving and integrated with your energy system.
5. Consciousness.
6. We can have a spiritual experience where we feel present, vital, clear, and purposeful.
7. We can feel spiritually uplifted.
8. Someone or something beautiful can "take your breath away" or "make your heart skip a beat."
9. Singing, speaking, praying, dancing can all be an expression of spirit energy.

What does it mean to have a broken spirit?

When I was 12, my parents took me to the zoo. I noticed one of the monkeys lying on the ground behind the glass with his eyes open. He was lifeless. They say that the eyes are windows to the soul. His light was dim. He was sad. He looked defeated, as if he lost his desire to live. Have you ever seen a wild animal in a cage like this? One that was taken from the wild and imprisoned. One who's been there long enough for the life force to drain out of their body. It can happen to us as well. We can become a prisoner of our mind and if we're there long enough we give up trying to be okay and the light in our eyes begins to dim.

We've all seen those commercials of abused pets. Dogs tied out in the weather suffering. If you take that dog out of that environment and give him love and support his light will shine again. While he may have developed defense mechanisms or quirky behaviors, he will not look for people to blame or hold onto resentment. He will be able to live a happy life.

There have been times I lost the will to live and be happy. Times when I felt like that monkey in the cage, lifeless and detached. My light was dim. I see-sawed back and forth between anxiety and depression, worry and defeat. It took me to some dark places and dampened my spirit for sure. Sometimes it's challenging to find things to be happy about, to look forward to. We wonder: "What's wrong with me?"

At first, I blamed Paul, my friend who committed suicide, for my mental turmoil, but over time realized that I was the only one responsible for my life moving forward. That was a major turning point for me. If you blame other people for your struggles in life, it will keep you stuck. The minute that you decide to assume 100% responsibility for yourself in the now, a shift will occur.

I'm not saying that the people who've done you wrong in the past, who've caused you harm should not be held accountable. I am saying, regardless, you must take full responsibility for your life moving forward.

The only way to get your power back is to forgive yourself and anyone else you hold in your mind and heart as the reason for your suffering. Forgiveness is a process of self-love. It's not a quick fix and it's not for the person who hurt you per se. The Latin root of forgive is *perdonare* and it means, "to give completely without reservation." We must give ourselves love without reservation in this way. If we try to bypass forgiving and just get rid of the stress, anxiety and overthinking, it's probable that we'll disassociate from our body in some way. You might think: if I can only get rid of my stress and anxiety, I'd be okay, when actually stress and anxiety are giving us vital information about ourselves.

Chapter 6
Anxiety and Stress Are Not The Enemy

You are not broken. There's nothing wrong with you. Your mind and body are doing what they were designed to do. Your body reacts to what the mind perceives and tells it, either consciously or unconsciously. Your body receives this information via the central nervous system (CNS). This information can be misinterpreted. When you're not actually in a life-threatening situation, yet your body carries on as if it is, you will experience a disruption in homeostasis.

When your anxiety runs high, some part of you doesn't feel safe. This can be indicative of your inner child. The part of you that is emotionally wounded from something in your past. When your inner child is controlling the narrative of your life and making the majority of the decisions for you, it can create an internal battle. It's as if there's two people inside of you battling for control. One part of you may want to go out and experience life, go on a trip, look for a new job, but the inner child sabotages your efforts. Instead, you might choose to stay closer to home, play it safe and avoid too much social interaction.

There may be several different types of anxiety, but they're similar in that, overthinking, worry and fear causes a physiological response in the body. General anxiety disorder (GAD), which most people experience at some point in life, is when our thoughts are like a runaway train and we worry and obsess about the normal things in life such as kids, job, money, etc. Post-traumatic stress disorder (PTSD) is when you've experienced a traumatic event that has lasting effects. Social anxiety disorder is when we get overly concerned about being in public or interacting in social environments. A panic attack may come out of nowhere, but something most likely triggered it. No matter what kind of anxiety we experience, we feel as though our life is threatened.

A perceived threat sets off a chain of events. Hormones are released into your bloodstream charging your system like a coiled spring, so that you can jump into action. This is known as the Stress Response, an automatic response turned on by a threat to a person's well-being. This is your innate intelligence at work to protect you. The problem is, you are most likely not in any real danger, but your body acts as if it is. People are living their lives in a heightened state of survival reacting to the constant barrage of stimulation from news, social media, screens, pings and dings and notifications. In today's world, especially in America, this has become a normal way of life, but it's not the natural state of a human being.

<u>The Stress Response (Sympathetic Nervous System Response):</u>
A built-in reaction that quickly, efficiently and automatically prepares the body to:
Fight: fight for your life
Flee: run for your life
Freeze: hide or freeze for your life

All vertebrates react to a perceived threat in a similar way, because our ancient survival system takes over. When the Stress Response is triggered, your body goes through a rapid systematic physiological change based on a "perceived threat."

Whether or not you actually are in danger is the real question to ask, because your body reacts even if it "thinks" it's in danger. These signals can come from merely thinking about something. In other words, you think yourself right into the stress response. In fact, this is the primary reason people experience anxiety and stress. They believe that something bad or life threatening is going to happen to them, but in the moment that thing is not actually happening.

One time my cousin and I were camping in an area of California known for bears. She had already set up her tent and went to sleep early. I stayed up late and was in the middle of setting up my tent in the dark. There were signs all over the park warning us to: Beware of Bears. While I had my arms full with my sleeping bag, pillow and toiletries I swore I heard a growl. I remember the hairs standing up on the back of my neck. Suddenly, I felt something grab onto the sleeping bag string. I jerked it back. I thought "Oh shit it's a bear."

It felt like a bear was pulling on the other end. In my mind, I was in a tug of war with a bear. A surge of adrenaline shot through me. I shrieked and pulled so hard on the sleeping bag that I fell backwards onto my cousin's tent. Her tent collapsed and I landed on top of her. For a few minutes we froze in dead silence. There was no bear, no threat, nothing wrong at all. The elastic string had gotten caught on the corner of the picnic table. When I pulled on it the picnic table moved and made a noise, then the string got stuck on a branch that created a spring like effect like something was pulling on it. In my mind it was a bear. My cousin was fine and it's now a funny story that we tell at family gatherings and a great example of a perceived threat that wasn't real.

A perceived threat can be anything: a deadline, concern for a loved one, worry that you're going to run out of money, public speaking, even the constant thought that something bad is going to happen. It can become a pattern.

The stress response begins in the brain when the amygdala is triggered. The amygdala is the fear center. It's part of the reptilian brain, the ancient part of our physiology that is 1000's of years old. When the amygdala is tripped it sounds the alarm and begins a complex series of events: powerful hormones (adrenaline, cortisol, norepinephrine) are quickly released into the blood stream. You instantly enter a heightened state of awareness. Your pupils dilate, your heart rate, breathing rate, and circulation increase, and muscles tighten.

Here's a very important concept to understand. There are varying degrees of this response. Getting chased by a pit-bull is going to elicit a different level of action than making a deadline at work, however both may very well trigger the response. If we are in real danger, we of course want our Stress Response to function the way it was designed, increasing our chances to survive the threat.

The severity of a traumatic event often goes deep into the tissues of the body. The body remembers, but the body also doesn't understand time, so it can feel like a traumatic experience happened yesterday when it really happened years ago. This is one of the biggest challenges with post-traumatic stress disorder (PTSD).

Unfortunately, a few of my clients have been onsite during mass shootings. These are obvious situations when we want our body to react the way it's supposed to, with a heightened state of awareness and the ability to protect itself. It's the after affects, the PTSD that becomes the challenge. The thoughts and feelings that linger on after the initial event. Going back over and over what happened again and again can be maddening. Soldiers and military personnel struggle with this very phenomenon. In situations like these we need a way to interrupt these thought patterns often and a way to communicate to the body over and over that what happened is in the past. "For real change to take place, the body needs to learn that the danger has passed and to live in the reality of the present."[2]

If you think and worry about something enough, it can trigger your amygdala. In fact, even watching the news can flip this switch. If we are not in real danger, but the Stress Response is activated to any degree, it will increase our heart rate, tighten muscles, and so on and we may not even realize it.

If we don't have a way of turning off this mechanism regularly, we will experience discomfort, angst, confusion, and disarray in the body. It will affect our digestion, sleep, and the general maintenance within our cells. If this becomes chronic, not only will it drive

---

[2]Von der kolk M.D., Bessel, The Body Keeps The Score, 2014

us nuts, but cause wear and tear on our organs leading to disease or illness.

The moral of the story is: you can go through the motions of life quite normally yet be living in a constant state of anxiety and stress. A heightened Central Nervous System (CNS) that keeps the body on edge will eventually cause burn out and dysfunction. How can we spend more time in life in the natural state?

The Natural State

Picture a deer grazing on grass in a field. Suddenly, it hears a nearby car backfire on the road. In an instant it bolts into the safety of the thick forest and monitors the situation by standing still. When it realizes the threat is gone, it goes right back to grazing on the grass as if nothing happened. It returns to its natural state. The deer is not thinking about what happened or worried that it will happen again. It just goes on living in the present moment. The deer's stress response is intact and working as it should.

One of the major differences between humans and animals is that humans are capable of thinking into the past or future to elicit feelings in the present. This can work for us or against us. Grabbing for positive visions or thoughts about the future helps us to create or manifest our future. On the other hand, if we stew about a bad decision we made or an event that took place or how we handled something that already happened in our past we may be attracting more of the same. Despite not being able to change what happened, we continue to spend time and energy mulling it over and over creating a thought pattern. This is a form of self-inflicted abuse or punishment. These reoccurring thought patterns become anxiety.

What's the connection between stress, anxiety, and depression?

The word anxious is derived from the root: *angh-* meaning painfully constricted or pain, which is how we might describe what happens in the chest during a panic attack. *Anxiety*: apprehension caused by danger, misfortune or error.

Anxiety can seemingly come out of nowhere. It can be triggered by something someone says, a scent, or even hearing a song on the radio. We call this the stressor or a trigger. Something that flips the switch. We may or may not be conscious of what triggers our anxiety. Maybe your boss tells you that if you don't hit the sales mark by the end of the month, your job will be in jeopardy. Now you can't sleep, because you can't stop thinking about how to make more sales and what an asshole, he/she is. The warning is the stressor, your constant worry is the anxiety. You might say that anxiety is prolonged stress, keeping the body in a perpetual state of fear. This can become a pattern that people get used to, even addicted to. Some people are so used to living with anxiety that when they don't have anything to worry about, it feels foreign. They may unconsciously look for things and people to worry about and are often labelled a worrier.

Stressor —> stress response —>worry —> anxiety —> depression.

Low bank account—>I'm in danger—>What am I going to do?—>Can't find a job —>Shut down.

In other words, your body's intelligence is working against itself even though it's functioning the way it was designed and programmed. It's being misinformed and reacting to that misinformation. Stress and anxiety can, therefore, perpetuate a dissociative mechanism (a separation of mind & body). You cannot think your way out of it. When you try, it perpetuates the very thing you're trying to get rid of and it becomes maddening and exhausting, which can lead right into depression.

Depression literally means the state of being pressed down or a sinking of the spirits. Anyone who deals with chronic stress and anxiety is susceptible to depression. We can only fight for so long, before our spirit breaks and we feel deep sadness and or grief. It's exhausting fighting against the body's defense mechanisms. Eventually, they resign and give up the fight. We call this depression. This is why people who are depressed seem to have no energy. It can be like handing in our own resignation. However, sometimes depression is nothing more than the body demanding deep rest. It's been fighting to maintain status quo for a period of time that it may need to be restored with a few days of rest and recovery.

Just as some stress can be good, a short lived shut down can also be beneficial as long as we make it good, consciously. We might need a down day or two in order to re-boot our system, get in touch with our feelings, process, integrate and come out reinvested in our path forward.

I teach several retreats per year designed for people to drop their defenses and get in touch with the root of their anxiety and pain. The truth of their situation. People from all walks of life come to learn how to love themselves unconditionally and leave with a renewed sense of themselves. They walk away lighter, brighter, and with a daily practice that gives them instant access to their spirit-self. The complete opposite of stress and tension.

It's when we are taken over by and not in control of our down time that is debilitating. Depression can be sneaky and seductive. It was for me. I justified my own self-loathing and self-medicating, which can easily lead to addiction.

Here are some questions to contemplate or journal about: What is at the root of my anxiety? What happened in my past that I cannot shake? What am I afraid of experiencing in the future? Where or what am I hiding?

The common denominator for stress and anxiety is not feeling **safe.** Stress triggers thoughts, worries, and past experiences of times when you did not feel **safe.** Childhood trauma, adult trauma, difficult times that provoked similar feelings of being out of **control and unsafe.**

Our programming or conditioning is based on our past, our childhood, our development, our experiences. This means that our perception drives the response, especially in situations that are not actually life threatening. Over time, this compounds on itself. It adds up. We may or may not notice our body reacting to our thoughts. We get worried that something is wrong, the stress of something being wrong creates anxiety and we are in a cycle that is hard to break. Chronic stress and anxiety creates confusion about what to do. In other words, you're living in a state of mind that lacks clarity and truth. The truth about whether you're in real danger or not. When we react to what our body is responding to, it can be difficult to know what to do.

To break this cycle, you must restore:
- Clarity (truth)
- Control (emotional intelligence)
- Safety (body/mind)

How?

The simple answer is, feel more. Chronic anxiety, stress, depression have some common denominators: fear, pain or hurt. Nine times out of ten there's emotional pain that can also manifest as physical. People who struggle with emotional pain often fluctuate between feeling numb, afraid, shame, angry, hurt, lonely, and finally grief. We must allow ourselves to feel our way through to what's lingering at the bottom of the pile, grief. Our emotional body has layers like an onion. As we peel back layer after layer: pain, fear, anger, sadness, we'll eventually get to grief. Grief is a force of nature and in many ways beyond our understanding. When we get to grief, compassion also arises and it's the compassion that we need for ourselves and others. Compassion is nature's equalizing energy, because it allows us to be with suffering, whether it's our own or someone else's.

Grief is complex and sometimes confusing. It does not always have to do with death. We can even experience grief years after we suffered a loss. It can be buried and often is. Grief is how our mind, body and spirit tries to integrate and understand life and loss, past and present. It's also a reminder that we are mortal. We experience grief when we have lost something, whether it's a loved one or a personal loss, such as our innocence or even the loss of control. Grief begets grief.

Many people suffer some sort of loss in their childhood or adolescence. It could be anything from the loss of a loved one, a traumatic event or maybe they had to take on a major responsibility at a young age. Maybe for whatever reason you were not able to have a "normal" childhood. Maybe you had to grow up and assume some responsibility that was out of your control. While the other kids were out playing, you had to care for a family member or members. Sometimes in life we disregard our own feelings to care for others to survive. Life presents all kinds of loss, but we aren't always aware of how they affect us. Sometimes it isn't until we can thoroughly and deeply relax into our body that things begin to unwind from our body and nervous system. One of the reasons people have a difficult time relaxing is, because when they do the body begins the process of elimination. Digesting, processing, and removing waste products in the form of material as well as emotional debris.

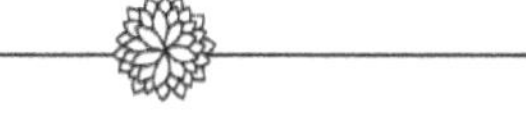

Chapter 7
<u>The Relaxation Response</u>

Stress generally has negative connotations, but a healthy amount of stress motivates us to complete tasks and pursue our passions. For example: writing this book was a huge project. I never wrote a book as in-depth as this, yet doing so gave me purpose. It took me over two years. It took discipline and vision. I had to put enough pressure on myself to get the job done without rushing and freaking myself out. I grew a lot in those two years. My voice, in the words I write, became more distinct and clearer. I also learned to finish what I started, which has become a new theme in my life.

Stress might take us out of our comfort zone, but it's also where we grow. My mom was 79 and my dad was 85 when they reluctantly got their first iPhone. My mom was understandably afraid of it. It stressed her out. She had not even dabbled in any kind of technology. She wanted nothing to do with it, but I knew that she could learn how to use it. It would give her immediate access to the rest of the family. I kept reassuring her until she finally broke through the fear and self-doubt. Now she's 82. She texts with emojis and GIF. She also has an iPad. She can navigate online quite well and feels connected to the extended family, which was especially important during the pandemic.

<u>Generally, there are four levels or stages of learning any new skill. This was originally formulated by Martin M. Broadwell in 1969, then Noel Burch made it widely accessible.</u>

1. Unconscious Incompetence: ignorance
2. Conscious Incompetence: awareness
3. Conscious Competence: learning
4. Unconscious Competence: mastery

The beauty of this, is that it applies to nearly everything and there's no time limit to each stage. I am currently between stage two and three in learning Spanish. I had to get over my fear of making mistakes or pronouncing things incorrectly. It's just part of the learning process. Once you understand and accept that it's through doing it wrong and imperfect that you actually learn. You can apply this to anything. You don't remember, but you fell many times when you learned to walk. You mispronounced words when you learned to read and speak. The truth is, you can learn almost anything if you're willing to fumble through not knowing and trust that you're in a process. There might be some initial challenges in the first few stages, but it's a good kind of stress.

Good stress is good for us. It brings excitement, but an overload brings fear and triggers the stress response. Dr. Fritz Perls, founder of Gestalt Therapy, said: "Fear is excitement without the breath." Meaning fear and excitement are closely related and breathing into fear can transform it into excitement. The opposite is also true. When you hold your breath, excitement can turn into paralyzing fear. Just think of standing on the edge of a cliff ready to jump off with a bungee cord. Thoughts can keep us living in fear.

Everyone is different in this way and has a different threshold. People have their limits and it's important that you know yours, because when you go into overwhelm for a prolonged period of time it burns out the system. When you are stuck in your head with constant worry and anxiety it affects sleep, digestion, relationships and so on. When this becomes chronic it will lead to more serious concerns such as high blood pressure, lowered immune system function, inflammation and general dis-ease in the body.

In 1975 the late Dr. Herbert Benson, through extensive research, proved that you can turn off the Stress Response by turning on the Relaxation Response. He said, "The relaxation response is a physical state of deep rest that changes the physical and emotional responses to stress…it is the opposite of the fight or flight response." It's synonymous with what I call the Natural State.

Benson outlined the importance of repetition and daily mind/body practices such as mantra (repeating of a word or phrase), repetitive motion, and meditation and why they work.

While the Stress Response or Fear Response (flight, fight or freeze) turns on the Sympathetic Nervous System, the Relaxation Response turns on the Parasympathetic nervous system (rest and digest). This will bring you into your natural state, where the mind and body are at ease and you feel safe. They cannot be "on" at the same time.

As a mind/body clinician, Dr. Benson defined and proved what had already been taking place within human anatomy and physiology since the dawn of humanity. He actually taught people how to manually turn on the Relaxation Response as a model for self-care and healing. When we direct our attention to the mind/body bridge for a period of time we elicit a physiological response that clears the mind and calms the nervous system. This is a simple, straightforward concept. It has been clinically tested and proven to lower: stress, anxiety, hypertension, cardiac arrhythmias, pain, insomnia, allergies, PMS, menopause symptoms, infertility and boosts your immune system.[3]

Current research continues to prove what Yogi's and monks have known and practiced for thousands of years. Training and integrating the mind/body/spirit resets or initiates healing.

The Breath is the Bridge Between The Body and Mind

While moving the body is important when it comes to integrating it with the central nervous system, conscious controlled breathing is paramount. This is a spiritual practice. Again, the Latin root word for spirit is spiritus, meaning: to breathe. The breath brings spirit to the mind and body. Of course, it does. While you can go days without food or water, most people would not last 90 seconds without taking a breath. It's the one thing we cannot go without. The breath is literally our life force. It's the bridge that connects the mind to the body and the body to the heart. Working with this bridge gives us the opportunity to feel more, not less.

---

[3] Herbert Benson M.D., Relaxation Response, 2001

54

Feeling more allows us to process and integrate our past and present experiences in life. Furthermore, breathing gives us direct access to our nervous system via the Vagus Nerve that runs through the diaphragm (breathing muscle). The Vagus Nerve is like a superhighway sending parasympathetic response signals from our brain, down the neck, into our gut and heart. Conditioning and massaging the Vagus Nerve through conscious active breathing is the central part of our mind/body/spirit practice.

Chapter 8
The Whole Body Breath

The very first thing you did when you emerged from your mother's womb was take a profoundly deep inhalation. Most likely the very last thing you'll do is exhale. Between your first inhale and last exhale is your life. The breath itself is therefore the most powerful healing instrument that we have, because it affects all the systems of the body and is immediately accessible to all people. Practicing how to breathe in developmental ways will not only greatly contribute to your overall wellbeing, but directly link you to the systems of the body that regulate and control thoughts, emotions, heart rate and immune response. Your breath is the link to reality itself.

There are generally only two types of breaths: unconscious breaths and conscious ones. In our everyday life, thankfully, we do not have to think about breathing, it's automatic and involuntary. It happens completely on its own. These unconscious breaths make up the majority of the breaths we take throughout our life. They take place all day every day no matter what you're doing. Bringing some awareness to how you're breathing throughout the day can be life changing. For instance, make sure that you breathe through your nostrils, rather than your mouth, most importantly on the inhalation. Also, catch yourself when you're holding your breath.

This often happens when we're stressed or overthinking. To be clear, I am not suggesting that you become obsessively aware of every breath all day. Not only would that be difficult, but you'd most likely not be able to perform the many tasks that give your life purpose and meaning. I am simply making the case for a daily breathing practice, which all by itself will increase awareness to how you breathe in general.

Conscious breathing is voluntary. Conscious breaths immediately heighten your awareness and connect you to your body. There are two types of conscious breaths: **passive and active**.

The **conscious passive breath** is when you're aware of your breath, but you're not controlling it in any way. There's connection to it, but you're not engaging it. Some people call this watching or observing the breath. You feel the rise and fall of your chest or belly and notice the air moving in and out.

The **conscious active breath** is dynamic, because it involves thought and action. This is vital to mental health. "When we follow the breath, the mind will be drawn into the activities of the breath."[4] If you move the breath consciously for a period of time thought patterns, stresses, worries, and mental disturbances will begin being dismantled. Depending on your focus and duration of active breaths thoughts may dissolve completely. You will not be able to think in any well-formed way when your full attention is on a more sophisticated breathing pattern.

Some breathwork techniques need your undivided attention in order to physically coordinate your

---

[4] TKV Desikachar, Heart of Yoga, pg. 56

breathing muscles to control volume, duration, speed, and so on. This is extremely helpful for mental health, because it draws your attention off of your worries and concerns and dials them into your life support system.

When you focus your attention on just breathing, it takes you inward rather quickly. When you keep your attention riveted on and in control of your breath cycles for an extended period of time, the mind lets go of thought patterns. The longer and more attentive you apply a breathwork technique, the more your thoughts will dissipate. I mean that within a breathwork session and over the course of several days of practice strung together. All **conscious active breathing** does this to some degree, but there are specific ones that clear the mind quickly, efficiently and completely. This will have an accumulative affect over time.

*Please refer to Appendix A in the back of the book for a complete list of the Seven Sacred Breaths, when why and how to use them.

The following breathing technique takes precedent over the others, because of the impactful nature of the technique itself. It's called **Ujjayi Pranayama.** Ujjayi means the victorious one and is the primary breathing technique recommended for any and all Hatha Yoga, Vinyasa Yoga and Asana (yoga postures and movements) in general, unless you have a contraindicated condition.

<u>An Important Note On Yoga</u>

Ask a variety of people what yoga is, and you will get as many answers. Much of the yoga taught today has

58

become diluted and fragmented. It has become more fitness based rather than a spiritual practice. I want to be clear about my interpretation, understanding, and experience in the Great Tradition of Yoga brought forth through Professor Tirumalai Krishnamacharya, widely known as the father of modern Yoga as we know it today. Yoga practice is to fully participate in life reality as it is given, as you are when you begin a Yoga practice. It must be adapted to the individual based on age, body type, health condition, personality and culture or belief system. There's no special place that you are trying to get to, but rather celebrate and accept your present condition. Traditionally, Yoga was taught one to one or in small groups, because the Yoga teacher's job is to help the student cultivate their own Yoga practice. One that they can enjoy on their own. The teacher is not above or better than the student, no matter what posture, education or level of "spirituality," they seem to be in. There's no hierarchy or place to ascend to. They are equals.

Over the past 25 years, especially, yoga has become even more standardized than it once was. Teachers and studio owners market yoga as physical fitness and more often than not teach the physical alignment of the body before students learn how to breathe properly. This has led to an overemphasis on physical prowess, movements, postures, stretching and so forth. However, flexibility, strength, and other physical attributes are merely byproducts of a complete Yoga practice. Yoga is first and foremost a spiritual practice. As I have re-iterated on purpose, the word spirit comes from the Latin spiritus, which means to breathe. The primary focus in a Yoga practice is the breath, more specifically Ujjayi Pranayama.

Without the breath life does not exist, so a breath centered practice is not only logical, but serves as the bridge between the body, brain and mind, as well as the heart of the individual. The asana (postures and movements) are done for the breath, not the other way around. This is a clear distinction from the vast majority of yoga being taught in America and abroad. Most of which is missing the foundational principles.

Someone's ability to touch their toes or bend in a certain way is a poor indicator of whether or not someone is making progress in their practice. A far better way to gauge headway in Yoga practice is to consider the relationships in one's life. From the relationship you have with yourself to all the people and things in your life. As you begin to understand and embody this distinction through a daily practice, you will be on your way to dismantle thought patterns and emotional trauma. Thoughts and physical symptoms that are associated with the root causes of stress and anxiety. This is why Yoga is the hope for humanity. Not as a cure or to fix a problem or attain something, but rather as an appropriate response to the conditions, speed and uncertainty that has become modern life. As a way to accept and participate in your own miracle of consciousness itself. Yoga practice is the key to actualize your gifts.

Ujjayi Pranayama: Building the Foundation

Ujjayi Pranayama is known as the Ocean Breath, because it mimics the sound of the ocean surf. Waves wash up on shore over and over in a soothing rhythmic action. All across the world water crashes on sandy beaches and rock cliffs where moisture lifts into the air.

These are sacred places, where the earth breathes. Where, for thousands of years people come to fish, eat, ride the waves, enjoy some respite, support and celebrate life. This too, is the nature of Ujjayi Pranayama: nurturing, calming, strengthening and stabilizing to the whole system. A recent study by the Centre for Integrative Medicine and Research in India found that: "Ujjayi Pranayama is effective in improving sustained and selective attention and reducing the state-trait anxiety of university students."[5]

It is the most dynamic breath that a human being can perform, because it is equal parts strength and receiving, meaning it is active on both the inhale (feminine) and exhale (masculine). This makes it balanced, rhythmic and meditative. It can be used and practiced all by itself or accompany movement. This breathwork technique gives you the most control at the strongest point in the body for breathing. In fact, Ujjayi Pranayama is the suggested breath to be used for all Hatha-Yoga, Vinyasa Yoga, and postural Yoga in general.

While it may be challenging to learn, you most definitely can learn it. In order to do so, you must recruit muscles that are not used all that much in everyday life, but it's well worth the time, energy, and focus it takes to learn it. In fact, when you practice Ujjayi Pranayama daily and become intimate with your breath, it will have a profound effect on your body and life. I've never taught breathwork to anyone who regretted it. If you choose to practice it regularly, it will serve you for the rest of your life.

---

[5] Parajuli Niranjan and Pradhan Balaram, 2/1/22, Effect of Ujjayi on Students Attention and Anxiety.

Generally speaking, most people have a weak diaphragm muscle. Out of the hundreds of muscles in the body, the diaphragm and heart muscle are easily the most important since they link us directly to our life support system. In other words without them, we could not sustain life even for a minute. Therefore, it's logical to condition the diaphragm muscle through a deliberate breathing practice as self-care and self-love.

Let's dive into the meaning of Ujjayi Pranayama. **Ujjayi** means the victorious one. **Prana** means: "that which is infinitely everywhere"[6] or energy that is everywhere. "**Ayama** means to stretch or extend and describes the action of pranayama." [7] Ujjayi Pranayama, therefore, means the victorious one who engages with and extends that which is everywhere. In this way, Pranayama balances our prana or the energy inside of the body with the energy outside of the body. This has profound implications.

The opposite of prana coming into the body is: **apana,** debris or that which is exiting the body. When there's an imbalance of prana and apana, it can disrupt systems in the body. Many ailments including mental disturbances, anxiety, depression, fatigue could be an indication that more prana is outside of the body than inside or vice versa. An example of this might be when we give too much of our attention, energy, care, worry etc. to something out of our control. We consciously or unconsciously allow our own vital energy to dip down, leak out or be diluted.

---

[6] TKV Desikachar, 1995, Heart of Yoga, Pg. 54
[7] TKV Desikachar, 1995, Heart of Yoga, Pg. 54

Emotions have a direct effect on our breathing. When we experience fear, our breathing will be stifled in general. If we're grieving, we might have trouble inhaling. If we're angry our exhale will be obstructed. Worry causes shallow breathing or worse we unknowingly hold our breath. Our emotions are directly connected to our breath and give us vital information. When we have enough prana moving through the inside of the body, we feel grounded and content. Too much prana inside and we might feel agitated or excited. Therefore, we can affect change and create balance in our system just through conscious breathing.

<u>How to activate Ujjayi Pranayama:</u>

Note: It's recommended that you consult with your physician prior to Ujjayi Pranayama. Contraindications include, but are not limited to: heart condition, blood pressure issues, pregnancy, breathing or lung disease. Do not perform Ujjayi Pranayama or bandha when your stomach is full.

The following instructions can be done in steps over time. It's important to consider that implementing Ujjayi Pranayama will likely feel and sound strange. I promise that this kind of participation with the energy in your body creates a deep connection with reality itself. I have broken down the technique and learning process into four steps. I recommend reading all the way through this chapter then go back and apply the instructions. Remember, in the previous chapter I outlined the four stages to learning any new skill. It's normal to experience awkwardness and uncomfortableness in the beginning, do it anyway. I literally taught my parents who are both in their 80's how to breathe Ujjayi Pranayama in less than five minutes. All you need is concentration and curiosity.

Step 1

Begin by whispering. Whisper a sentence three times in a row. Make it louder each time. It can be anything, how about: "I will practice deep breathing every day for one week." Whispering will get you in touch with the muscles in the throat that are capable of restricting the air flow, which is what creates the whispering sound. Get in touch with that sound and the feeling in the throat. A similar sound is made when you fog up a mirror or a window with an exhalation. The same sound is created when you use your breath to fog up your sunglasses, it creates a haaaaaaaa sound.

Step 2

Take a deep, yet relaxing breath in through your nostrils until you feel that the lungs are full, pause, then open your mouth and from the back of your throat breathe out haaaaaaaaaaaa. Take your time and do this 3-4 times in a row to activate the muscles of the larynx. Go slow. Practice making the exhalation long, slow and smooth.

Step 3

Breathe in through your nose, pause for 1-2 seconds, exhale through your nose while maintaining the same throat sound. Don't try too hard. It can be subtle at first. This will challenge you, but you can do it. You breathe in and out through your nostrils making the haaaaaa sound in the back of your throat on the exhalation. It might help to place two fingers at the hollowed-out notch at the throat between your collar bones.

<u>Step 4</u>

To refine the breath further, try to make the throat sound on your inhalation as well as the exhalation. Again, it can be subtle. Breathe in and out through your nostrils only, continuing to make the throat sound. You may have to gently press the tongue against the roof of your mouth just behind the upper front teeth to stabilize the back of the tongue/glottis area. This will help you to restrict the air flow in and out at the throat. Clear your throat as needed.

Even though the breath moves through the nostrils first, it passes through the throat area before making its way down the trachea (bronchial tube) and into the lungs. This will challenge you both mentally and physically, which is why it works, so well. Concentration is key. You must focus your attention on an area of the body that you most likely don't think about much in addition to applying the technique itself. Make a commitment to learning it! Out of anything that you can learn to do better in life, breathing is a sure bet. It's one thing that will change everything, I promise.

<u>Four Parts to One Breath Cycle</u>

One full breath in and out is a breath cycle. A breath cycle actually consists of four parts: 1. inhale, 2. pause, 3. exhale, 4. pause, then repeats. In everyday life, pauses may seem non-existent unless you're really paying attention. When we practice our breathing or do our Yoga, we want to be deliberate and in control of all four parts of the breath cycle. This alone has a positive effect on your entire system. It's completely normal, even suggested to make the exhale last a bit longer than the inhale, especially when first learning to breathe this way. It's easier to make the haaaaaa sound on the exhale and helps to condition the muscles being used. Over time, you'll want to try to make the inhale and the exhale the same in duration, volume and care.

Inhalation (1):

In Ujjayi Breathing, we create resistance by restricting the air flow at the throat, then we breathe against the resistance. Since the diaphragm muscle contracts only on the inhalation it has to work harder to draw the air in and is therefore strengthened. Interestingly, we don't suck air into the lungs, rather the diaphragm creates a vacuum and air is drawn in. One way to think of Ujjayi Pranayama is strength training for the diaphragm muscle and a massage for the Vagus Nerve. Remember, the Vagus Nerve gives us direct access to the Central Nervous System (CNS), which is responsible for turning on the *Relaxation Response,* so we can drop into our natural state.

Pause (2):

When we pause the breath after the inhale, we continue to condition and tone the diaphragm muscle, increasing its ability and receptivity. Holding the air in keeps the diaphragm muscle contracted, so we have both increased resistance and maintain a longer duration of muscular contraction. This gives us more control and will be very useful when we coordinate the breath with body movements. You do not need to pause the breath for very long, a second or two at first will be fine.

Exhalation (3):

Interestingly, the diaphragm muscle relaxes on the exhale and has no ability to push air out. In order to empty all the air from of the lungs, we use the abdominal muscles. In fact, the abdominals initiate the exhalation and follow it all the way to its end. By contracting the abdominals in toward the spine and slightly upward we squeeze out all of the remaining air from the lower lobes of the lungs. This is actually the reason why the Heimlich maneuver works well when someone is choking, and their airway is blocked. When you quickly and firmly pull someone's abdominals in and up, the leftover air in the lungs forces whatever is blocking the airway, out. We call this lower abdominal contraction, Uddiyana Bandha. Of course, we are not using a quick, firm force when implementing the bandha, but rather a slow steady engaging of the musculature.

Pause (4):

On the pause after the exhale, the abdominals are held in for a second. This is a perfect set up for the next inhalation, which will allow the chest and upper thorax to fill first, then the abdominals can relax as the belly area fills last.

Bandhas

Bandha means to bind, lock or seal. It involves contraction and cooperation of muscles in three primary locations in the body. The pelvic floor area between the pubic bone and tailbone down to the anus is called Mula Bandha or root lock. You might know this as a kegel exercise, but it also involves contraction of the anus muscle. The lower abdomen area is Uddiyana Bandha, which initiates the exhale. The third is in the neck/throat area and is called Jalandhara Bandha. Implementing Jalandhara elongates the cervical spine of the neck. For our work together, we will primarily focus on Uddiyana and Mula Bandha.

<u>Bandhas serve three main purposes:</u>

1. Help protect the body, especially the spine. 2. Aid in directing toxins and debris towards the fiery heat building breath of Ujjayi Pranayama. 3. Purify the energy centers and channels in the body.

When practicing Ujjayi Pranayama, we use Uddiyana Bandha, which assists the exhalation by contracting the transverse abdominal muscles and squeezing them inward. We pull the lower belly in towards the spine and slightly up. The abdominals initiate, follow, and complete the exhalation. This will help to empty the lungs completely. When performing the Bandhas, it's important not force or try too hard. Mula Bandha grows naturally out of performing and understanding Uddiyana Bandha. They work together.

<u>Practicing Uddiyana Bandha:</u>

1. Take a deep breath in through your nose to fill your lungs.
2. Pause.

3. Contract your abdominal muscles or squeeze the lower belly in as you exhale the air out.
4. Pause.
5. Repeat.
6. Try doing four or five consecutive breaths.

That's it! It's a coordinated muscular effort done on the exhalation.

Ujjayi Pranayama and Bandha Creates The Foundation For Yoga Practice

Postures or asana help to create bandha naturally. Moving the body in various ways aids bandha application. For example, when you bend forward from a standing position the movement itself initiates the exhalation and compression of the lungs. Therefore, whenever you bend forward it should always be with an exhalation.

Being With The Breath:

Use the throat sound that you learned from above to the best of your ability. Start by drawing the belly in. Hold it in as you begin the inhalation. This can be subtle and not meant to be a struggle. This will allow you to fill the lungs from the top down. Fill the chest, upper back, rib cage, then the belly. This will allow the inflation or expansion to take place in all directions: top to bottom, side to side, front to back. The rib cage will telescope up and away from the hips. The upper thorax and ribs themselves will stretch out to the sides and the sternum will grow forward while the upper spine pushes back. You can think of it as a two part process, fill chest and upper back first, then belly and low back with the same inhalation. A deep breath in has a wonderful way of standing the body upright and lifting your spirits at the same time. In fact, a deep inhalation can naturally adjust vertebrae, which is what a chiropractor does.

There are a few places to feel the expansive quality of the inhalation with your hands to help you navigate and be with the breath:

- Place your hands on your upper rib cage just below your chest muscles near your armpits. When you breathe in deeply, you can feel the ribs lift up and expand outward into your hands.

OR

- Place your right hand on your sternum (center of chest) and your left hand on your lower belly. When you breathe in deeply, the hands will separate slightly as the chest lifts up and away from the hips and the belly softens and fills. Here's where you can practice filling the chest first, then the belly. Once you've inhaled to capacity hold the breath in for about (1-2 seconds).

Remember the transverse or lower abdominals initiates and follows the exhale. Start the exhale by drawing the belly in while resisting the temptation to empty the lungs out all at once. Take your time pushing the air out slowly by using the throat sound to control the air flow out. Think of it as a tire under pressure with a small hole in it. The air leaks out slowly rather than all at once. Contract the abdominals in until you're empty. Empty from the bottom up. Pause the air out for a second or two. Now you're ready for the next inhalation. Repeat the same process.

This may sound like a lot, but there's no hurry to learn it. You can do it, but you must concentrate. Once you get the hang of it, it's quite natural. Anything worth doing will take time, focus and energy. I promise you with all my heart that this breath will unequivocally, absolutely, 100% change your life! It can't not work if you practice it. I have never ever taught this to someone who said that it didn't help them clear the clutter from the mind and revitalize the whole system. It's well worth learning and doing. This is what's missing from many yoga classes nowadays. If you already practice yoga, this is the breath you should be using.

Allow your practice time to be a safe space. Make a commitment to yourself to start with 10 minutes per day. This is quality time that you spend with yourself, learning and growing. It will take your attention off of your worries and clear your mind.

Growth is never comfortable, but always worth it. Growth occurs throughout life regardless, breathing with it allows us to integrate and actualize it. Breathwork balances the energy in our mind and body by removing obstacles or that which does not belong.

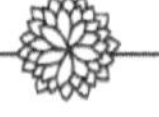

Chapter 9
Intimacy With Life

From the 5th to the 14th Century, Yoga flourished as a practical means by which people from all walks of life could actualize and share ideas as part of daily life, done in a non-hierarchical way before power structures, religions or authoritarian governments were established.[8] Mark Whitwell

In the 17th Century the word intimacy was used to mean sexual intercourse. While it can still evoke this same sentiment today, the meaning has expanded to include trust, connection and plutonic relationships of all kinds. In fact, many people have sex, but are not intimate. The adjective *intimate* comes from the Latin term *intimus,* meaning innermost or deepest. The French had originally spelled it: *intime.* If we extrapolate the origins of this expansive, often misunderstood word it means to spend time with or share our deepest, innermost feelings and thoughts. To become intimate with oneself and our life, we direct our attention inward, *in to me.*

Many indigenous cultures around the globe acknowledge the seven directions: east, south, west, north, above, below, and the seventh one turning

---

[8] Mark Whitwell, 2004, *Yoga of Heart*

inward. This is synonymous with many Yogic and religious scriptures. The body itself is our temple. Yoga is the ancient technology of intimacy and provides the gateway into our temple, riding on the magic current of the breath.

<u>Yoga: The Technology Of Intimacy</u>

Humankind needs intimacy more than ever. Yoga in this way is a healing modality and greatly underutilized today. In a world that has gone viral with material and information, intimacy is the missing link to heal people and the planet. Intimacy, first with our own body, breath, and our true nature, which then translates into all other living beings and the material world including the earth. We are not separate from nature; we are nature itself. This is at the heart of Yoga. Yoga is the ancient technology that allows us to intelligently integrate and actualize the reality of life within and around us.

I'm not talking about modern yoga that has been over duplicated, standardized, and made popular by branding it through the fitness and fashion industries. Not the yoga that has been commodified, codified, and often stripped of its essence. Again, I want to make a clear distinction here between fitness yoga and the Yoga of intimacy or participation. What many people are calling yoga nowadays is basically a physical fitness or stretching class often bordering on gymnastics. Many modern yoga classes are often taught by popular, in shape teachers who have crossed over from the dance, modeling, fitness, and fashion industries. They tend to lean more into the physical fitness side of yoga or asana with challenges and goals. I'm not saying that these classes don't have some merit or useful benefits, especially if you enjoy them. I do, however, want to draw a line in the sand. I want everyone to feel included and supported with an actual Yoga practice no matter what your physical ability is when you begin.

A Yoga practice that is right for you and guided by the heart of Yoga principles found in the next chapter, as well as in appendix A in the back of this book. These principles will help you meet yourself exactly where you are at the time of your practice session without the need to try hard to attain some "better" or deeper body position. Yoga is then accessible to all people regardless of your body type, age, health condition or belief system.

This is the Yoga of intimacy that was passed down through caring, considerate teachers to be shared with all of humanity. It's not just for flexible or fit people. I'm talking about Yoga for each individual based on when you choose to become intimate with your own life. A practice that is right and appropriate for you, no matter your weight or personality. A practice that can be applied to your life situation no matter what that is.

Yoga in this way is very practical. It is the means by which to embrace and shape your miracle of life every day. When we are with our breath, we become intimate with our own body and mind. It is our God given right to be intimate with the self, to care for the self: body, mind, emotions, and spirit.

When we tap into the nurturing and creative force of life by being with our body and breath, we assimilate the ancient intelligence and wisdom that is already flowing within and around every cell of our being. If that's not God, nothing is. To know thyself, our body of truth, our *innermost,* is direct interaction with source itself. The journey to get somewhere more enlightened or better by following thought patterns of men in power is bogus, because it denies the truth and extraordinary wisdom that we already are.

When we are intimate with our body, breath and relationships of all kinds we feel more, we see more clearly. We naturally develop more compassion, patience, and tolerance. This intimate, loving endeavor begins with the most important relationship we have, with self. From there it naturally flows into all other relationships, especially with your partner or spouse.

Somehow the word "sensual" has become associated with sex and therefore religion. Originally, a sensual experience was a heightened physical ability, usually associated with pleasure. As we become sensual, we are more sensitive, which mainstream society has imposed a negative connotation. Being sensitive or attuned is a gift. I'm not suggesting that we allow ourselves to be taken completely over by our feelings, but rather be honest with them. The actions we take or don't take when we get real with our feelings has more to do with emotional intelligence than sensitivity.

The beauty of becoming more sensual and sensitive with your own body and breath, is that it goes with you everywhere. Whether you're at work, listening to a friend, helping an elder or connecting to your partner.

The practice of intimacy with self can and should translate into great sex. Sex in this way is a healing endeavor! You can most definitely charge up your love life with a deeper intimate connection with your own body and breath. Yoga. I mean this alone could be reason enough to cultivate an actual Yoga practice, but certainly not the main focus of this book.

I am rather making the case for you to take some time every day to align your-self with source by controlling (mind and brain), your breath (spirit) in coordination with the rest of the body (physical) using movements and positions (asana) to transform your overanxious mind (Chita Vritti) into peace and harmony (shanti).

When you hold your attention on this interaction and interplay for a period of time daily, something wonderful happens. The mind first sets the path of the breath, then follows the breath into the body. As it does, it releases patterns of attachment to everything outside of itself and surrenders to the body. The mind becomes the body and releases the need to "do" or "get" or "pursue" anything at all. When this occurs, you will experience a profound rest and perhaps a great relief as you go from thinking to doing to being. Some time will go by without worry, cognitive thought patterns, or the constant urge to be busy. It might only be for a minute or two at first. Consistency and lengthening your daily practice can extend those minutes. When these conditions have become manifest, meditation arrives naturally. Thoughts slow down, maybe even stop. The general belief is that you ascend or transcend to some better place, but what actually occurs is not transcendence at all, it's the shedding of everything that is not you, so that you can align to and fully experience the source energy that is always coursing through you.

You may drop so far into yourself, into the intelligence that beats your heart every day, that you once again experience the bliss, wonder, and great mystery of life itself. Once you participate in this state, your reality becomes enjoyable, because you're finally fully in the present moment. It's not meditation as in some other higher or better state of consciousness, but rather our natural state, which is nurturing and loving. It's really love that we're all searching for, and we've been conditioned to believe it comes from the outside in.

If we nurture love from the inside out, happiness becomes less illusive and more readily available, because peace is already our natural state. The more we live in our natural state, the more we can relate to everything and everyone. Healthier relationships with one another and the earth itself is what the world needs. That's why we say, Yoga is the hope for humanity.

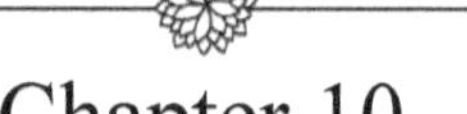

Chapter 10
Dancing With Your Miracle: Yoga Practice

T he heart is a highly sophisticated organ. It beats over 100,000 times per day. It takes less than a minute for the heart to pump blood around the entire body. The heart also has the ability to produce and secrete hormones and neurotransmitters that regulate Heart Rate Variability (HRV). This refers to the heart's ability to regulate itself with tiny fluctuations that cause it to beat faster or slower depending on what messages it receives.

Science, religion and medical research continue to delve into the function, ability and relative emotional states that affect the heart. Recent studies indicate that Heart Rate Variability (HRV) can be improved with Yoga. In fact, breath training has a direct effect on HRV. The reason this is so important for anyone with anxiety, stress or trauma is because Yoga will over time help you to be able to self-regulate.[9]

An actual Yoga practice is a personal endeavor that not only turns on the Relaxation Response but increases the GABA neurotransmitter that is scientifically proven to lower anxiety and depression.[10]

---

[9] Bessel Van Der Kolk, 2014, The Body Keeps The Score p.p. 268-271

[10] Boston University. 2007, May 22

Your Yoga is your Yoga influenced by what you can do (sadhana) and what you believe. The beauty of Yoga as technology is that no matter who you are, with some coordinated effort, you can begin to dismantle the obstructions that keep you from experiencing a profound sense of self love, joy, peace and belonging.

As you do your Yoga practice there will be a certain amount of time that passes when your thoughts will be fleeting at least or absent altogether at best, instead of completely formed and active. They will be broken apart and undeveloped. When you create the time and space to drop into yourself to have some time without anxious thought patterns and old stories, even if it's just for a few minutes, it becomes very healing. When you consistently, daily, practice bringing yourself into that healing space, it expands. It provides the three most important things you need to live your life peaceful and happy: safety, clarity, and control of your own well-being, including your thoughts.

Not all yoga is created equal, nor are all teachers educated to understand anxiety, trauma or how psychology and neuropathy are connected. There are plenty of yoga instructors that can show you how to do Yoga postures "correctly," how to align your musculoskeletal anatomy to feel the "stretch." However, there are fewer actual Yoga teachers who truly understand the significance of, or even how, to facilitate you past your insecurities, past your social mask, past your to do lists and into the "neutral zone." A place within yourself without worry, fear, or the feeling of carrying the weight of the world. This is where you align with source or spirit, the Natural State. The Natural State is like space, where there is zero gravity.

Think of a rocket ship. In order for a rocket ship to enter orbit where there's zero gravity it must have enough thrust and direction to push through the resistance of atmospheric pressure, friction, and gravity. Once the rocket reaches orbital velocity it can turn off the engines and float through space. At this point, the astronauts can look back and see the magnificent beauty of planet earth. The gigantic bodies of blue water, the expanses of green continents that have no borders, and the rise of mountains spread across the planet.

In Yoga practice, we create a steady burn by breathing deep and free. We move our body into the reality of the present moment and our worries about the past and future begin to drop away. Sometimes sensations will arise in the body and trigger a memory or emotion. We allow those emotions to come through. We give space for it, but stay with what is happening in the now, our breath and body movements. This takes concentration, technique, and effort, but it is available to everyone. It's as if new information is being installed into a system that is already prepared to accept it. You can think of it as an update for your magnificent internal computer.

Before we add more movement and create shapes with the body (asana) by applying different angles to the limbs and torso, it's important to understand that the movements and positions provide context for the breath itself. As we reach, bend, twist, and lengthen muscles, we create more space for breathing. Our primary focus is on the four parts of the breath cycle and how they relate to the position of the body. The postures create a map with avenues and angles for energy or prana to follow. We want to give enough attention to filling and emptying the lungs without getting caught up in the trap of being overly concerned with how far we can stretch or bend the body.

This is one of the ways that the western mindset of conquering and bullying the body has negatively influenced yoga. So much of the American version of yoga has come from a projected and manipulated mindset. This occurs when we use will and force to manipulate the body instead of building rapport and relationship with the subtle nuances of the breath. Trying hard is often synonymous with getting a good workout, feeling accomplished and good enough, but often misses the larger invocation. Trying too hard can actually cut off the flow of energy.

We are not bending the body to our will, we are listening to the body and taking part in its wonder. That doesn't mean that we aren't challenging our body when it's appropriate. It just means that we want to prioritize the importance of listening and receiving while we implement the movements and postures. In this way there's no end point, no certain pose that lets you know that you've arrived. No place that you're trying to get to. Remember you are already here as a miracle of life. When Yoga is done as participation only, all movements and postures simply reinstate this message of wonder and gratitude. In essence we are learning how to better communicate and feel within our anatomy and physiology. Taking into consideration both the physical and energetic fields. Wherever blood flows and nerves run, energy is involved. It's that simple. We are merely taking part in what's already happening in life. The following pillars and principles make Yoga entirely your own.

<u>Understanding The Four Pillars of Yoga Practice:</u>

1. <u>Asana or Body Postures, Movement & Form:</u>
We move the body in different ways to access different parts of the body. The asana or body positions are like streets or pathways we create for the energy from our pranayama (breathing) to flow. In a well-designed practice, energy is evenly distributed to all areas and parts of ourselves. From mind to muscles to bones to nerves and organs, our whole system is refreshed. There is a logical sequence (vinyasa krama) of postures to take for each of us based on our unique life experience and condition of our mental and physical body.

2. <u>Pranayama or Breathwork:</u>
There are several different kinds of Yoga breathing techniques used for everything from asana (postures) to relaxation to cold water therapy to stimulating the nervous system. Please refer to Appendix A in the back of this book for the Seven Sacred Breathwork techniques, when why and how to use them. The breath is a key to our participation. Ujjayi Pranayama (Chapter 8) is "the" breath to use for asana (moving and stretching).

3. <u>Dhyana or Meditation</u>
Meditation is a result of our breathing and moving practice. Breathing and moving clears the mind chatter and worry from our mental space, then we can rest quite peacefully, naturally. Meditation must not be forced, but rather invited into our experience. It

literally arrives as a result of our asana and pranayama practice. Refer to Chapter 11.

4. Nature or Life in a Seamless Process

Our Yoga practice is the appropriate action for us to take to fully be with our life and our born reality. When we are intimate with ourselves, we become relatable to everything outside of us. Yoga is how humans process and integrate being human. As we care for ourselves in this way, we naturally want to care for others and the earth itself. We hopefully, will realize that we are, in fact, one! When Yoga practice becomes a daily routine of self-care and self-love as normal and natural as washing our face or brushing our teeth, it becomes easier to recognize ourselves in others.

The following is a complete general Yoga Practice for most bodies, ages and conditions. It is a non-denominational practice and can either be done in its entirety or broken up and done in parts. It is a template that guides you through both breathing and moving the body (Dynamic) and breathing while staying in the postures (Static). You can think of the practice as whole-body prayers. It should take around 25-35 minutes depending. It's important that you tailor the practice to your individual needs. If you're unable to perform a movement or posture, skip it and go to the next one. There's no substitute for having a good teacher to help guide, educate and keep you accountable for doing your Yoga.

What You Need For Your Yoga Practice: Preferably, a quiet place without distractions. Outside at a park is nice.

You can do your Yoga on a carpet or yoga mat or the grass. The important thing is to be on a non-slip surface, preferably barefoot. Yoga blocks can be helpful in certain poses for balance and height adjustments when using the floor for poses. However, the beauty of doing your own Yoga is that essentially all you need is yourself.

Your Own Yoga is powerful, practical, and healing every single time that you show up and do it. If you do your Yoga in the morning, it's nice to face East where the sun rises. These easy-to-follow **Heart of Yoga Principles** can also be found in Appendix A:

1. **The breath movement is the body movement.** When the body moves the breath moves with it. They become one. When you hold a pose (static), you allow the body to mold around the breath cycles. Give enough physical space to receive a complete inhalation then take up that space with a complete exhalation.
2. **The breath envelopes or encapsulates the movement.** It begins just before the movement starts and ends just after the movement stops. For example, the parentheses here: ((Movement)) indicate the breath
3. **The inhalation comes down from above, the exhalation rises up from below.** We receive on the inhale and give strength on the exhale. Together they are strength receiving.
4. **Bandha is the natural cooperation of muscle groups.** Uddiyana Bandha assists the exhalation by drawing the lower belly in and up.

<u>**Remember:**</u> On each **inhalation**, relax the surrounding musculature (shoulders, neck, face) to fill the lungs. This will take concentration and may even be counterintuitive, so give it time. When inhaling allow the rib cage to lift or telescope up to create more space between the ribs and hips. Be patient while the lungs inflate to completion. Pause for a second. On each **exhalation**, engage your lower abdominals in and up. During the practice, in different positions or postures, you'll move and breathe (Dynamic), then, stay and hold a particular stretch or posture (static), and breathe.

<u>Standing Poses:</u>

Begin with your eyes open and a soft, fixed gaze on a point in front of you.

Samasthiti: Standing at Attention and Reaching Up

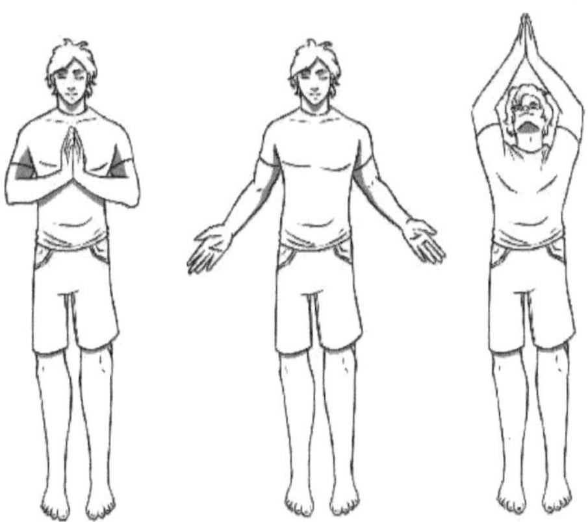

<u>Intention:</u> Honor the direction above where the inhalation comes down from.

<u>Benefits:</u> Lubricates shoulder joints, stretches neck, back and chest musculature, expands lung capacity,

elongates and stimulates vertebrae. Spiritually uplifting.

<u>Position and alignment:</u> Begin standing upright with feet approximately hips width distance apart, knees are soft, not locked. Eyes focused forward and slightly down. Hands are relaxed, fingers together in front of the heart in a prayer position. Alternatively, arms and hands hang down alongside of the body. You should be sturdy, comfortable and attentive, not rigid. This could also be done seated.

<u>Movement and Breath Pattern:</u> Inhale as you sweep the arms and hands up and around, so the hands meet again above the heart. Pause the breath and the movement. The arms could be straight, or the elbows slightly bent. If possible, look up as the hands go up, without straining the neck. Begin the exhale and return the hands to the starting position. Pause the breath out.

<u>Simplified:</u> 1. Inhale, sweep arms and hands up. 2. Pause at the top. 3. Exhale hands return to starting position. 4. Pause.

<u>Duration:</u> Repeat 4-7 times.

<u>Helpful Hints:</u> When you reach up, lift and expand the ribcage with a slight back arch by filling the lungs all the way. It's as if you're drawing a large circle in the air around the head and heart with your hands.

<u>Static Movement and Breathing:</u> The last time you reach up, stay. If possible, keep the hands touching above the heart in a prayer position for 3-5 Ujjayi breaths. Return hands to starting position in front of heart. Rest the breath.

Standing Forward Bend: Uttanasana

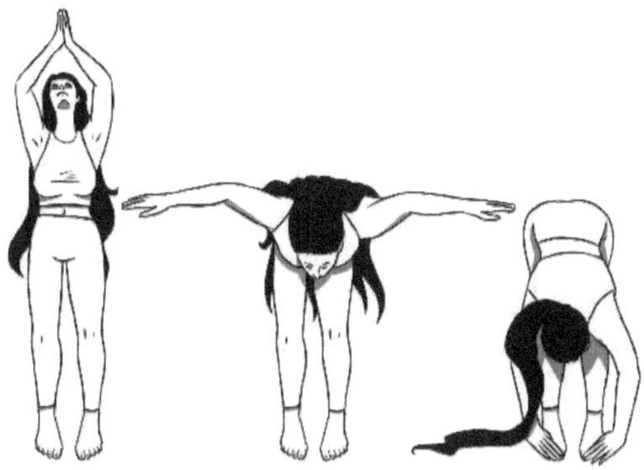

Intention: Bow down as a gesture of gratitude and recognition of the direction below, where the exhalation arises from.

Benefits: Stretches the entire backside of the body, flexes the spine, lubricates vertebrae, stimulates organ function and digestion, increases blood circulation to the brain and face, soothes nervous system. Activates spatial awareness.

Position and Alignment: Stand upright, feet hips width distance apart. Knees are soft, not locked. Hands in a prayer position in front of your heart or hanging alongside body.

Movement and Breath Pattern: Inhale to sweep the hands up and over the heart. Lift the eyes up and align the hands above the heart. Pause. Exhale to bend forward and touch the floor if possible (no forcing). Pause the breath out for 1 second. Inhale as you rise and reach back up.

Simplified: 1. Inhale, sweep arms and hands up. 2. Pause at the top. 3. Exhale, bend forward to touch the ground. 4. Pause at bottom. 5. Inhale, reach back up to the sky. 6. Repeat.

Duration: Complete 4-7 times.

Helpful Hints: Lead with your sternum or heart as you bend forward. Do your best to bend from the hips first, then allow the back to round as the spine flexes. Relax neck and head at bottom. You can bend the knees to accommodate the movement. On the way back up lead with the arms.

Static Movement and Breathing: On the last forward bend, stay down. Grab onto your feet or ankles and breathe 3-5 more breaths. Relax the musculature a bit to fill the lungs on the inhale. Pause. Engage abdominals to naturally go deeper into the stretch on the exhale. After the last exhale, pause. Inhale leading with the arms to rise and reach up. Pause. Exhale and return to starting position.

Rest body and breath for 7 seconds but stay attentive.

Standing Side Bend: Parsva Urdhva Hastasana

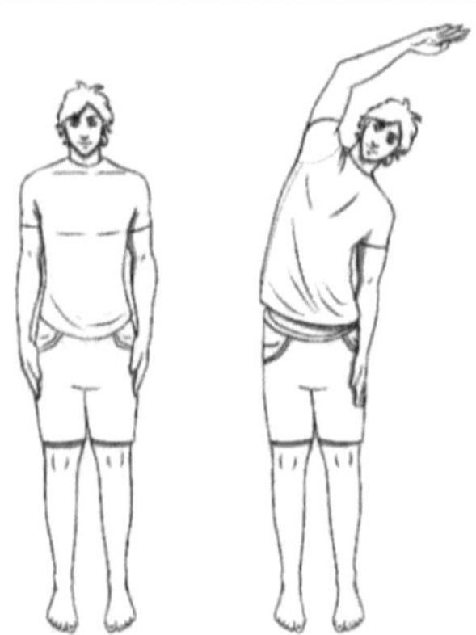

Intention: Yoga is the union of opposites. Honor all directions as they converge inside of you.

Benefits: Stretches lower back, neck, abdominal and hip muscles, keeps spine supple, increases range of motion in shoulders.

Position and Alignment: Stand with feet close together. Look forward. Either touching or a few inches apart for stability. Your arms are hanging down alongside body.

Movement and Breath Pattern: Inhale to lift right arm up and over, side bending to the left. The left-hand slides down and presses against the left thigh for stability. Gently, allow the left ear to drop towards the left shoulder. Pause. Exhale and return to starting position. Pause. Inhale and do the other side. You can look up at the upper hand if it agrees with your neck, otherwise look straight ahead and allow your head to bend to the same side.

Simplified: Inhale, reach right arm up, bend to the opposite side. Pause. Exhale return to start. Inhale, repeat on the other side.

Duration: 4-7 times on each side.

Helpful Hints: Take your time filling and emptying the lungs. Avoid overstretching or pushing past the breath.

Static: Inhale, bend to one side and stay for 2-4 breaths. Return to starting position on an exhalation. Repeat 2-5 breaths on other side.
   Return starting position and rest, but stay attentive with a soft gaze on a point in front of you.

Parvritta Trikonasana: Standing Twists

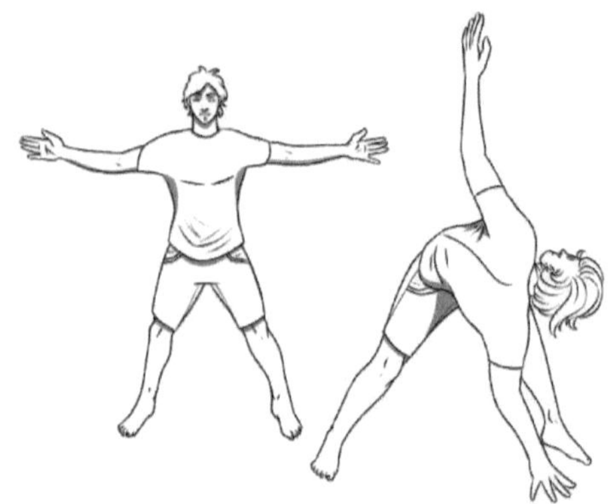

Intention: Keep an open heart as you bend and twist through life.

Benefits: Restores suppleness to spine, stretches and strengthens back, hips, core, stimulates organ and digestive function.

Position and Alignment: Stand upright with your feet wide apart (approx. 3-4 ft.) and parallel. There's not a set distance for how far apart your feet should be. You want them much wider than your hips, but not so wide that your balance is off. Avoid locking your knees. Hold your arms straight out, level with your shoulders like a five-pointed star.

Dynamic Movement and Breath Pattern: Inhale until you feel the chest lift and lungs fill, pause, exhale twist the torso to the left and bend forward reaching your right hand to the left foot area, pause. The chest stays open through the movement. Inhale rise back up arms out wide, pause, exhale twist and bend forward, left hand to right foot area, pause. Inhale rise back up to the starting position.

Simplified: Inhale. Pause. Exhale bend forward reaching right hand to left foot. Inhale to starting position. Exhale, reach left hand to right foot. Repeat. Duration: 3-5 times on each side.

Helpful Hints: Engage abdominals on the way down. Your hand can reach down to anywhere near the opposite foot. Remember the breath begins before the movement starts and ends after the movement stops.

Static Posture and Breath Movement: The fourth time that you bend forward and reach to the opposite foot, stay in the twist and breathe 3-5 more pranayama breaths. Even out the weight on each foot. Let the posture and musculature soften a bit on the inhalation, engage the abdominals and twist a bit more on the exhalation. Maybe you can straighten the knees more on the exhale, lean forward or backward to adjust the posture and feel more action in the body. After a while this becomes intuitive. Inhale back up, pause, exhale do the other side.

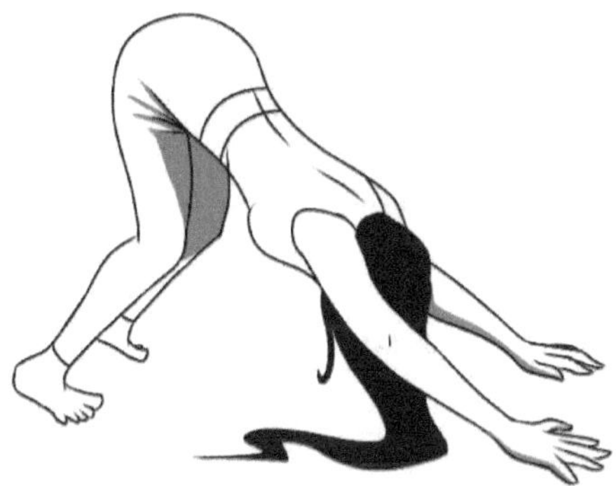

Transition: From Standing to Kneeling Poses:

From standing in Samasthiti (upright and attentive), inhale to reach up, pause, exhale to bend forward, pause, place the hands down on the floor (bend the knees as needed). Once hands and feet are on the floor walk the feet back until they're 3-4 feet away from your hands. Lift your butt or sitting bones high. This is Downward Facing Dog Pose- Adho Mukha Svanasana. You can also have the knees slightly bent here and the heels may or may not reach the floor. Take 3-5 Ujjayi Breaths. Then come down onto your knees and rest.

<u>Kneeling</u>

Balasana: Childs Pose

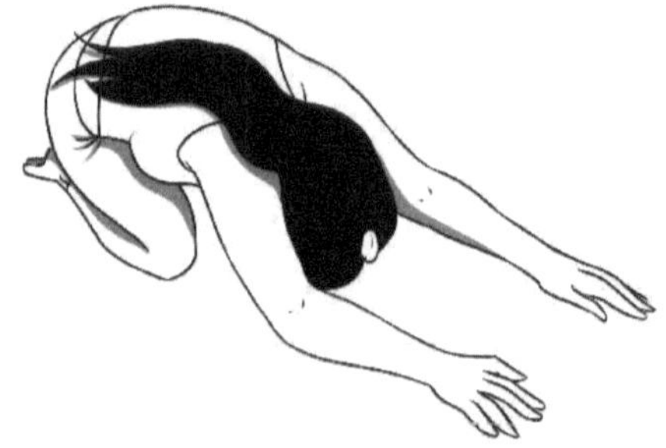

<u>Intention:</u> Come down to the earth, coil around and nurture your heart and mind to remind us of our innocence and purity.

<u>Benefits:</u> Emotional support, grounding, stretches lower back and hips, restful, sedates the nervous system.

<u>Position and Alignment:</u> From your downward facing dog pose, gently bring your knees down to the floor, separate your knees wider than your hips, sit your hips back toward the heels. As you do leave your arms stretched out. Rest arms and your forehead on the mat. Soften and surrender here.

<u>Simplified:</u> From hands and knees position, separate knees wider than hips, sit hips back towards heels, rest head on your mat.

<u>Duration:</u> Rest for 10-20 seconds.

<u>Helpful Hints:</u> Generally, this is a resting pose. If your head doesn't reach the floor, use a folded towel, pillow or yoga block to rest it on.

<u>Dynamic Movement of the Spine:</u>

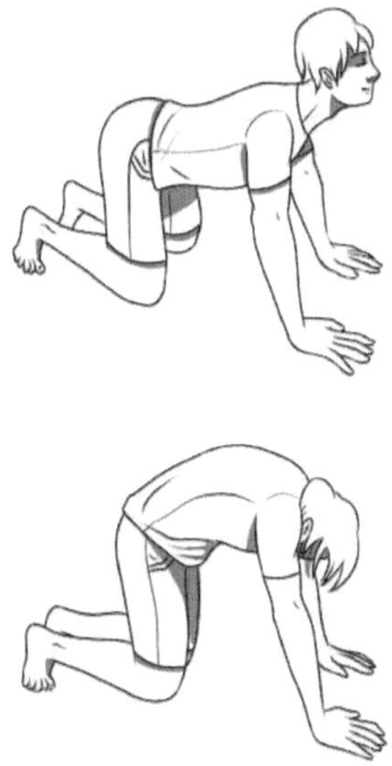

<u>Intention:</u> Mimic the movements of a child crawling by flexing and extending the spine to keep the body supple and mind sharp.

<u>Benefits:</u> Keeps the entire spine supple, lubricates joints, increases neural pathway proprioception, increases lung capacity.

Position and Alignment: Begin on your hands and knees. Align your shoulders elbows and wrists. Hips over knees. Hands open and active, meaning you're gripping the floor with your fingertips like claws. Toes can be curled under, stretching bottoms of feet or rest the tops of feet on floor by pointing toes toward the wall behind you. Your eyes can be closed here.

Movement and Breath Pattern: Remember, the movements are initiated by the breath cycles. Inhale, look forward, arch the back, stick your butt out. Pause. Exhale, round the back and sit back into your Child's Pose stretching your back. Pause. Inhale return up to the hands and knees position. Repeat.

Simplified: Inhale arch the back, pause, exhale round the back and sit into child's pose, pause. Repeat.

Duration: Arch the back and round the back into Child's Pose 4-10 times.

Helpful Hints: Take the time to fill the lungs and expand the rib cage in all directions, then contract the lower abdominals in and up on the exhalation. Whether you need a rest or not allow the body to land in this new position to recalibrate a new relationship with earth and gravity. Avoid forcing the stretch.

Transition: Lie down flat on your belly.

Lying Down

Salabhasana: Locust Pose

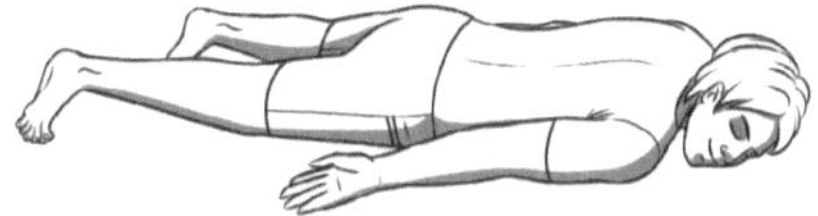

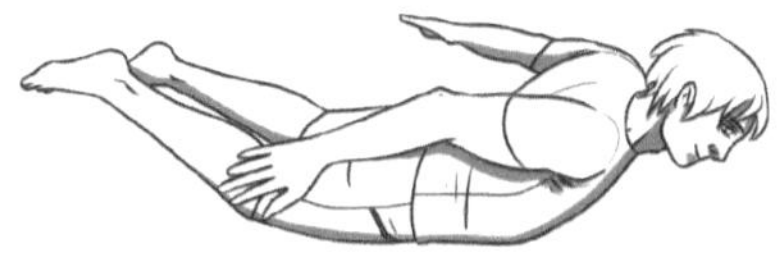

Intention: Bring your heart, brain, and hips close to the earth to ground thoughts and fears.

Benefits: Strengthens entire backside of body, especially spinal muscles, strengthens diaphragm muscle.

Position and Alignment: Lie flat on your belly, arms alongside the body, palms down. You could place a folded blanket under hips to provide some extra padding. This is a straightforward movement for stimulating contraction of the spinal musculature.

Movement and Breath Pattern: As you inhale press your hips down into the floor and lift your chest, arms and legs up. Keep arms and legs straight. Look downward at the floor. Pause. Exhale and return the chest, arms and legs to the floor.

Simplified: Inhale arch up, pause, exhale, lower down.

Duration: Do 4-7 times.

Helpful Hints: As you lift up, draw the shoulder blades back towards the spine and focus your gaze down and forward.

Static Posture: The last time that you arch the chest, arms and legs up, stay up for 4 full breaths. Exhale on your way down and rest. This will be challenging but avoid struggling by adjusting how far you go up. Make sure you're receiving a full breath in when you come up.

Transition: Either place your hands down on the mat under your elbows and push yourself into downward facing dog or onto your hands and knees for a few breaths. Roll over onto your back.

Bridge Pose: Setu Bandha Sarvangasana

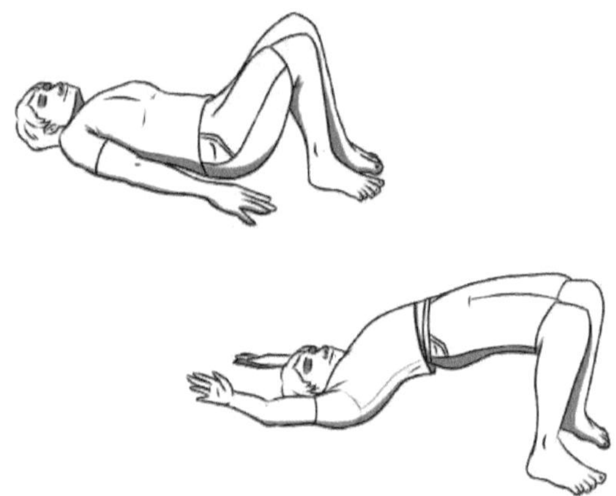

Intention: Support from the backside opens the front of the body to prepare us for the future.

Benefits: Creates space for organs, strengthens back of the body and legs, stretches hip flexors, stimulates the spine, and heart rate.

Position and Alignment: Lying on your back face up with your knees bent, feet flat and parallel, arms resting alongside your torso, palms down. Keep knees approximately hips width distance apart.

Movement and Breath Pattern: As you inhale lift the arms up and over head, press your hips up toward the ceiling, and the chest toward the chin producing a back arch. Pause. The exhale returns the arms and hips slowly back down to the floor. Pause. Repeat.

Simplified: Inhale lift arms, hips and chest up. Pause. Exhale return to starting position.
Duration: Repeat 4-7 times.

Helpful Hints: Feel free to adjust the feet and shoulders as you come up. Take your time to fill and empty the lungs completely without struggle. Ease up on the musculature as you breathe in all the way. As you exhale lift hips higher.

Static Posture with Breath: On the next round use the inhalation to lift the arms, hips and chest up. Stay up for 4 or 5 full breaths. **Optional:** Bend your elbows and press them into the floor alongside your torso while pressing the hips up and back arched. On the last exhalation come down and rest 10-20 seconds. Place your right hand on the chest, and left hand on your belly. Feel for your heartbeat. Stay connected to your source for 10-15 beats.

Transition: Rock your knees over to the left then right, slowly twisting back and forth 4 or 7 times.

Apanasana: Knees Into Chest Pose

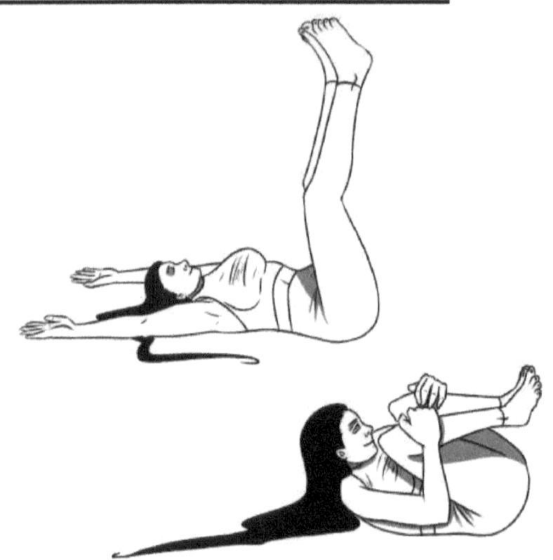

Intention: Apanasana means wind relieving pose, so don't be surprised if you let out a fart or two. Apana also means outgoing or removal of waste.

Benefits: Stimulates organ function, especially digestion, aids in emptying lungs, stretches and flexes the spine, hips and low back.

Position and Alignment: Rest with your legs hovering straight up above hip/belly area and your arms above your head on the floor. Alternatively, if you need to, bend the knees slightly and hold the legs with your hands.

Dynamic Movement and Breath Pattern: As you exhale use your hands or arms to pull both knees into your chest squeezing all the air out. Pause. Inhale as you straighten the legs back up toward the sky and the arms above the head. Pause. Repeat

Simplified: Inhale straighten legs and arms up, pause, exhale squeeze the knees into your chest emptying all the air out.

Duration: Repeat 4-7 times.

Helpful Hints: You could lift your head off the floor as you squeeze the legs into the chest. Take your time filling and emptying. Pause for 1-3 seconds after each inhale and exhale.

Static Posture With Breath: Inversions are when the legs or the majority of the body is held higher than the heart. Lift your legs up and stay for 1-2 minutes. It might seem like a long time, but it's so healthy to hold the legs higher than the heart. It should not be a struggle. If you need to, use your hands to help hold the legs up. When finished return your feet to the floor. Place your right hand on your heart and left hand on your belly. Tune into your heartbeat. Rest for a full minute.

Transition: Grab onto your legs and rock yourself up and back a few times to a seated position.

Ardha Matsyendrasana: Seated Twists

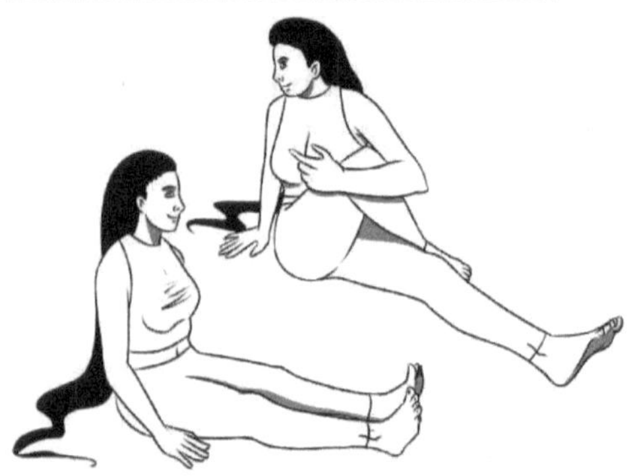

Intention: Twist the spine for a worried mind and create more space for nerves and energy to flow.

Benefits: Tones and stimulates spine and organs, stretches hips, soothes nervous system, relieves stress and anxiety.

Position and Alignment: Sit upright with your back straight and both legs straight out in front of you. Bend right knee, step up and over left leg or alternatively, place the foot in front of the right hip. Sit tall with chest lifted, engage core. Hug the bent right leg with your left arm. Place your right hand on the floor behind you for support. Repeat on opposite side.

Static Posture With Breath Pattern: Inhale to lift and lengthen the torso upward. Pause. Exhale and engage your abdominals and twist to the right looking over right shoulder. Pause.

Simplified: Inhale grow tall, pause, exhale engage the twist.

Duration: 4-5 breaths on each side.

Helpful Hints: Soften the pose to receive a full breath in. As an aid for less flexible people, you could place a folded blanket under your butt, so that your hips are slightly lifted (approx. 1"). Also, slightly bending the straight knee can help you sit taller.

Transition: Straighten legs out in front of you.

Paschimottanasana: Seated Forward Bend

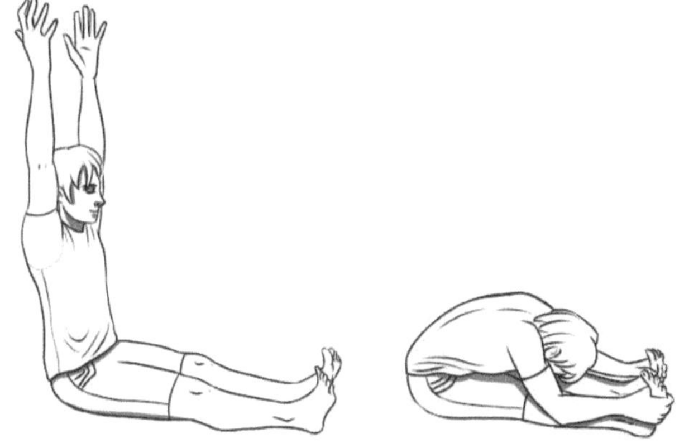

Intention: Reverence to life. Paschimottanasana means westward facing intense stretch, because traditionally you'd be facing east, the back of the body would be facing west.

Benefits: Intensely stretches the back of the body from the heels to the head, compresses and stimulates all vital organs, calms the nervous system.

Position and Alignment: Sit upright with your legs straight out in front of you. Arms resting alongside body. Notice the two bones that you're sitting on. Try to sit up on the front edge of your "sits" bones instead of rolling off the back edge. You may have to bend the knees a bit. Feet should be active.

<u>Movement and Breath Pattern:</u> Inhale deeply as you reach up, lift chest and rib cage. Pause. As you exhale, bend forward reaching to your feet. Bend from the hips first, keep your chest lifted and eyes focused forward on the way down, then allow the spine to round as you lower your head.

<u>Simplified:</u> Inhale reach and lift sternum up, pause, exhale bend forward, pause.

<u>Duration:</u> Repeat this movement coordinated with your breath 4-7 times.

<u>Helpful Hints:</u> You can place a folded blanket under your seat (approx. 1"). Bend your knees as needed to help you sit more upright.

<u>Static Posture:</u> On the last repetition that you exhale and bend forward on, stay. Breathe 4-5 more full breaths. Ease the posture to receive a full breath in, pause, engage belly to go deeper on the exhale. When finished, inhale and reach back up, then rest with your hands in a prayer position in front of the heart for 10 seconds. Enjoy the calm.

Transition: Move right into upward plank or reverse tabletop pose.

Purvottanasana: Upward Plank Pose

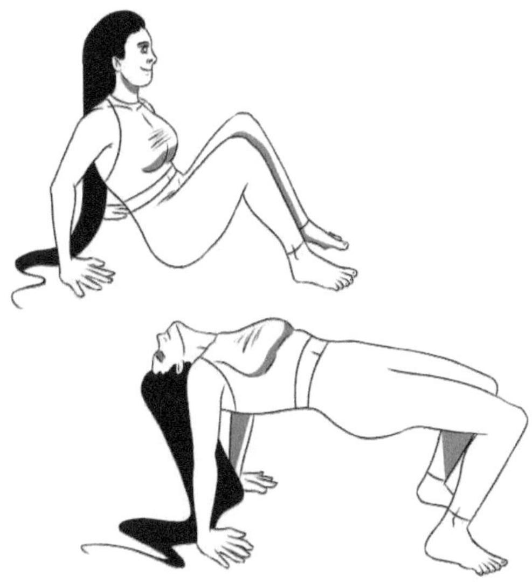

Intention: Explore new possibilities of movement and support with curiosity and trust.

Benefits: Stretches the front of neck, chest, shoulders and hip flexors. Strengthen glutes, legs and back. Develops unique relationship with earth.

Position and Alignment: Place hands flat on the mat just alongside or just behind the hips, shoulder width distance apart. Fingers pointing forward or slightly out to the side. Bend your knees and place feet flat, hips width distance apart. Eyes focused forward.

Movement and Breath Pattern: On the inhalation, push hands and feet down into the mat while pressing the hips and chest up toward ceiling creating a table with the front of your body. Pause at the top. Exhale and return to starting position. Pause. Repeat.

<u>Simplified:</u> Inhale, press hips up, pause, exhale lower hips down.

<u>Duration:</u> 3-5 times.

<u>Helpful Hints:</u> You can either keep looking straight forward or gently release your head back, so that you're looking behind you.

<u>Static Posture:</u> On the last repetition up, stay up and breathe 3-5 full breaths.

Transition: Return to a comfortable seated position. Here you can sit in a cross-legged position on a pillow or cushion, so that your hips are higher than your knees. Alternatively, you can kneel with a yoga block or pillow between your ankles, under your seat or even sit in a chair if the floor doesn't work for you. Sit upright, but not rigid. Spine is straight, soften shoulders, neck, jaw, arms and hands.

<u>Seated Pranayama:</u> Alternate Nostril Breathing for a round of ten OR do The Rest Breath (Appendix A) After your seated breathwork rest for a minute or two.

Transition: Lie down on your back.

Supta Matsyendrasana: Simple Supine Twist:

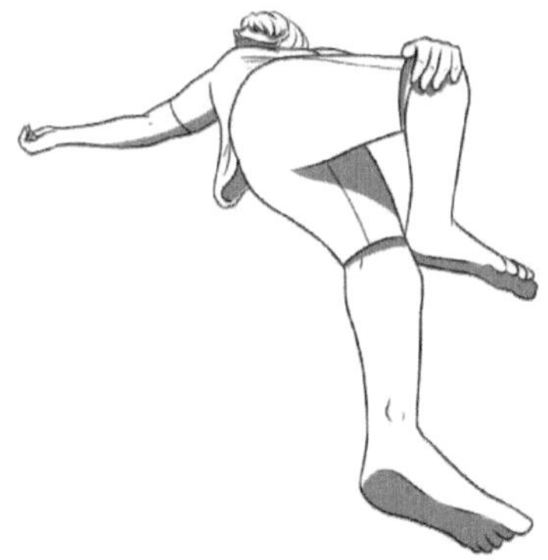

This is a transitionary posture preparing you for deep rest. Bend your right knee then bring it all the way over to the left side of the body. You may have to slide the hips over to the right a few inches before you make the twist. Leave both shoulder blades resting on the mat. Remain in the twist and breathe in a relaxing way for a minute or so, then repeat on the other side.

Intention: A final rinse and flushing of all that does not belong in this sacred miracle body.

Benefits: Releases low back and hips, naturally brings spine and vertebrae back into neutral alignment, detoxes organs and relieves tension throughout entire body.

Position and Alignment: Lie on back, face up. Bend one knee towards torso. Bring knee across the body until the hip on the same side lifts and stacks over the other hip. Rest.

Movement and Breath Pattern: Rest your breath and body in the posture.

<u>Duration:</u> Approx. 1 minute on each side.

<u>Savasana: Corpse Pose</u>

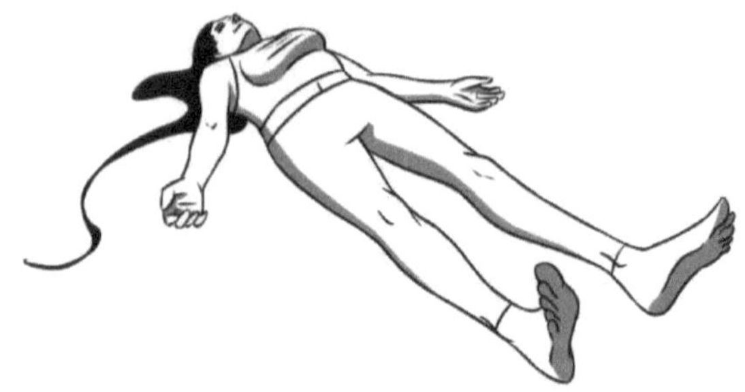

<u>Intention:</u> Surrender to Life.

<u>Position and Alignment:</u> Lie flat with your arms resting alongside your body. Turn your palms up. Close your eyes. Rest your breath and body completely. Be still. Meditation begins.
<u>Duration:</u> 3-10 minutes.

By now, the vast majority of your everyday thoughts will have fallen away or at the very least become fragmented.

Allow all body parts and muscles to soften. A nice way to enter this deep rest is to consciously, internally scan the body beginning at the feet. Move your awareness up the body releasing contracted muscles and any residual tension along the way. Pay particular attention to areas in your body that are chronically tight. For most people it's usually neck, shoulders and low back. From the feet to the ankles, shins, knees, thighs. Let your breathing rate slow down. Notice your hips, low back, belly. Feel the support of the earth beneath you, trust this. Relax your upper back, rib cage, shoulders. Continue to let go. Arms, hands, fingers rest. Head, neck, jaw, face release. Take notice of your heartbeat and any other sensations that arise naturally. Give yourself full permission to be with the rhythm of your heartbeat. If you feel emotions permeate to the surface, allow them to move through you.

This is the gift (Siddhi) of your breathing and moving practice. To *"Be"* without having to *"Do"* anything.

A deep Savasana is extremely nourishing to yourself as an organism. It's as if your built-in computer system is receiving an update from the universe, fixing glitches and bugs. The information that came through your effort of breathing, moving, and stretching is settling into your cellular structure. The beauty of this update is that it's 100% innate. The body's wisdom and intelligence does all the work. You set it in motion by linking the breath with movement, the mind to the heart and whole body, then be still and allow it to move on its own within you.

In Savasana, the mind lingers in the quiet. The noise of life becomes distant, like falling asleep on the beach. Some wonderful things happen. Throughout your practice of moving and breathing and bending and reaching and twisting and stretching, you open energy channels throughout the body called Nadis. Similarly, in Chinese medicine, the channels are referred to as meridians. These are real. Acupuncturists use needles to manually open areas that are blocked. They are separate from, yet connected to the blood and fluid systems in the body, which are connected to the body's electrical or nervous system. Let's not forget that we are mostly water and water conducts electricity.

In any case, a logical sequence of Yoga postures (Vinyasa Krama) also opens and clears obstructions throughout the network of channels. Healing is occurring all on its own. In Savasana, we rest with less obstruction of our energy flow. You may literally feel this buzz or vibration in the body while in Savasana. I hope you do, it's a special experience and often under appreciated. You know when you have had a successful practice when your body feels at one with the ground beneath you and your mind has let go of any agenda at all.

Here, in the quiet, is an opportunity that may not be available to you while you're in your "doing" life. With fewer thoughts, a quiet mind, less tension and resistance in the body you can communicate with your inner being, your true self. You can literally talk to yourself, be kind to yourself, the way you would speak to someone who you love and appreciate. You can say all the things that we like to hear from our loved ones, but perhaps don't hear enough. You can forgive yourself here. You can tell yourself how much you appreciate this body. You can unconditionally love yourself, your whole self.

While resting in Savasana place your right hand on your heart and your left hand on your lower abdomen. Take a minute to connect to your heartbeat. This heart has been beating for you since before you were born. Be with it for 10-20 beats. Notice the energy moving through and around you. This energy is always with you, but now you're consciously aware of it and bathing in it. When you feel ready, repeat these mantras. Remember you are speaking directly to your inner being or spirit-self.

1. Thank you.
2. I forgive you.
3. I love you.
4. You are a miracle.

Say them 3x each. Let each one land in your body and being. Rest completely for 5-10 minutes. You cannot unconditionally love someone else, until you love yourself. You cannot forgive someone else, until you forgive yourself. Make this an intimate part of your practice. You can also do this exercise upon waking in the morning or before you fall asleep.

<u>Savasana to Seated Meditation (Dhyana):</u>

With eyes closed, from Savasana roll over to your side and rest in a fetal position for a minute. This position itself is nurturing, reminiscent of when we were afloat in the amniotic fluid, safe and secure in our mother's womb. After a few minutes sit up-right comfortably. You can sit on a folded blanket to lift your hips higher than your knees. Sit as comfortably as possible. You can even sit in a chair with a back or lean against something. Once you're upright and settled, reconnect with your breath. Take one or two deep breaths then breathe easy. Let your belly relax.

Settle in and enjoy resting for three to twenty minutes. There's no time frame here. Just enjoy the moment for as long as it lasts. When you feel complete bring your hands together in a prayer position (mudra) in front of your heart and bow your head down as if to say Amen or Thank you or Shalom or Namaste or something that feels appropriate for you. Then, go have the best day ever, knowing that you're loved and that you belong. You are nature itself and the power of the universe lives inside every cell of your being!

Do this practice every day. Don't worry if you miss a day. Just pick it up the next day, don't make a big deal out of it. Creating a daily practice is not a perfect science, but the act alone communicates love to your soul. This is a process, and it may not feel great every time, but do it anyway. Get twenty-five practices under your belt and I guarantee that you will be in a different head and heart space than you once were. Every time you show up in the name of participating in your body and breath, you shed more of what no longer serves you and you bring in what nourishes your spirit.

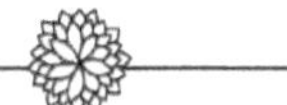

Chapter 11
<u>Meditation Naturally</u>

Sit down, shut up and listen! I first heard this phrase from an overwhelmed substitute teacher in fourth grade. We were bad kids that day, completely out of control yelling, screaming, throwing things around the room. In the midst of our chaos, we ignored the teacher's timid pleas to bring order back to the classroom, until suddenly, something wonderful happened. The sub lost her shit. Despite the fact that she was a petite older woman, she let us have it. From somewhere deep within her one-hundred-and-ten-pound body erupted a roar that could have rivaled a tiger.

"HEY! SIT DOWN! SHUT UP AND LISTEN!" At the very moment she roared, she flipped a desk over onto the floor. BOOM! Everything stopped. She had reached her boiling point and disdain for our behavior. It was beyond any expression of rage in public that I had witnessed up to that point. God knows my Italian mother could yell, but this woman's voice penetrated our little bodies. Silence fell on twenty kids in an instant. She had our undivided attention. We all sat down, shut our mouths, and listened very intently. She had redirected our attention off of our shenanigans and onto her. We felt her intention to establish control and order in the classroom. Once she had our attention she spoke quietly, yet clearly. She said,

"The next person who raises their voice or gets out of their seat will immediately go to the principal's office and we will call your parents. Am I clear?" she asked.

We all nodded. For the rest of the day, we were as quiet and attentive as little church mice lined up on a pew. Throughout the day, she subtly reminded us that there would be consequences for bad behavior. In other words, she held us accountable for our actions with certain conditions. I call this attention with intention.

That substitute teacher woke us up to our actual reality. While we were feeding off the emotions of excitement, we lost track of where we were and what was expected of us. We were acting outside of ourselves and out of control. We became part of the chaos around us.

From micro to macro, is this not indicative of where we are as a human race? Are we not being pulled outside of ourselves with other people's drama, excitement, media and chaos? Are we not swept up in constantly comparing ourselves to everyone else? The consequences of which, are wreaking havoc on our health as well as the health of our planet. This is not new. Yogi's, mystics, shamans, wisdom keepers, and Indigenous peoples have been sounding the alarm on this for hundreds if not thousands of years.

When our substitute teacher interrupted our frenzy and brought us back to reality, a major shift took place quickly. We came to our senses. We went from out of control to in control. From reacting to listening. From action to presence. From a wandering mind to stillness.

We became fully present. The teacher was then able to hold our attention on the tasks that we needed to complete throughout the day. This is mindfulness or the art of paying attention.

<u>Meditation Distinction</u>

Before we dive in, I'd like to draw a distinction in order to clarify the two overarching types of meditation.

There are many different expressions of meditation, from transcendental to guided meditations and visualizations to Zen Buddhist forms etc. However, there are really only two types of meditation: **passive and active**. Instead of trying to differentiate between the various constructs of meditation, I want to speak to the common threads of all passive or traditional meditation often referred to as mindfulness meditation which are to: sit with a quiet mind, increase awareness, be with yourself, expand and explore consciousness, and uncover inner peace.

Passive meditation means that you're not active or busy in your mind. You're not creating a future, visualizing or journeying to another place or time. You're simply "being" where you are. I like to think of it as **resting awake**. It is the practice of merely being present with your own breath and body and surroundings. Passive meditation is heartfelt and compassionate. This does not mean that thoughts and feelings are not occurring, it means that we don't have an agenda when we sit. We sit for the pure joy of being alive, like watching a sunset. The act of sitting or in some cases mindfully walking, is the art of being.

Conversely, there's a growing number of people who call being guided by and visualization or projecting or even manifesting, meditation. This has been coined "active meditation." It's when you're "doing" something. In this form the mind is active and busy while you're sitting still with the body. Your aim is to access certain feelings and thoughts in order to create your future. This falls into the category of manifesting or attracting things in your life that you want. I like to refer to this as queuing up the quantum field, because it's about creating your future.

This is a highly useful practice, but it's not the meditation practice I'm teaching or referring to in this manual. In fact, I believe that both types are powerful and useful, but learning to passively sit in meditation is a deeply nourishing way to accept your current reality before wanting to change it. In fact, when we learn to passively meditate first, we create a clear channel for whatever you may want to come next.

You can think of passive meditation as surrendering to the miracle of life that is already in you as you. The one we are currently living in the present.

From this point forward I will only be referring to passive meditation for our work together.

Meditation: the Gift (Sidhi) of Moving and Breathing

Meditation is to rest in our being-ness. It gives us an opportunity to become present with our current reality through paying attention. It's not that we're trying to remove our thoughts, but rather let our thoughts and feelings just be. It's true that if you sit long enough your thoughts will eventually fall away, but for most people, until that happens, suffering may ensue. For people new to meditation, it can be a miserable experience. When we sit in stillness, the body might stop, but the mind continues to manufacture thoughts. Trying to sit still and meditate implies that you're not actually meditating. Trying to meditate without preparing the mind and body can actually add to your mental anguish and suffering. Krishnamacharya, the father of modern Yoga and the teacher of the teachers said, "You cannot meditate, you can only make the conditions right for meditation to occur naturally."

The most efficient way to drop into yourself is to make the conditions right for meditation to occur naturally. In this way meditation is an integral part of the Yoga practice. Do your deep concentrated breathwork (pranayama), moving and feeling (asana) in direct coordination for some time (10-90 minutes). This will break up structured thought patterns. The mind literally follows the breath into the lungs. As your mind rides the breath into the body, thoughts drift away like clouds parting to reveal your inner sun. Here the mind becomes the body itself and you can just enjoy basking in the light of your own being.

Focused breathing and moving in a synchronized fashion does all the heavy lifting, so to speak, because your attention is deliberate and has sustained intention. It's as if the mind gets fatigued enough to let go. By the time you get to your (Savasana) at the end, you're ready to rest in this natural state of being. Now you can fully receive the gift of a seated meditation from your asana and pranayama practice. We go from moving meditation to being still in meditation. While you rest in this state, it's inevitable that at some point you will experience a oneness with the entire universe, because the entire universe lives inside of your own body as intelligence.

The four parts of our Yoga practice strung together in a seamless process disarms the nervous system and defense mechanisms. By doing so, you have access to and can communicate directly with your inner being or spirit self. By the very nature of your actions, you are transmitting: **safety, clarity, support and control of your emotional body. These are the pillars of peace and contentment.**

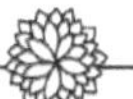

Chapter 12
The Truth Will Set You Free

How to shift from negative self-talk and thought patterns to a more positive, healthy attitude. The exercises at the end of this chapter along with your daily Yoga practice will keep you moving forward on the path of mental clarity and healing.

Have you ever wondered why some people see the world in a positive light while others look for what's wrong? Our upbringing, past experiences, and choices in life shape and mold us into adulthood. If we haven't learned how to look on the bright side or find a silver lining in dire situations, we might think that the universe works against us. When we believe that things happen "to us" instead of "by us" or "through us," we are living from a victim mentality. To change this, we must understand that the universe doesn't know the difference between what you want and what you don't want, it only responds to what your attention is on.

Things happen in life that are both out of our control and challenging to deal with, but this happens to everyone. I have never met anyone who didn't experience the highs and lows of life, yet these challenges or hardships do not have to define us. When the chips are down it's easy to fall into the trap of: "why is this happening to me?" The truth is "it" happens to everyone sooner or later. However, if you're in a pattern of "things happening" to you, you must upgrade your mental framework and take more control of your thoughts and emotions.

The question is not: what if something happens that is out of my control? The question is: when something happens out of my control, how will I deal with it? Will I react or take right action? Reacting is a knee jerk response, while taking right action is an appropriate mindful decision. The Bhagavad Gita outlines the importance of action and truthfulness.

We all have those self-defeating thoughts from time to time, but when negative self-talk is steady and constant, it's easy to drift into troubled waters. No one wants to feel as if they're being kicked around by outside forces. No one wants to be negative or feel bad unless there's a payoff. If any part of your identity is wrapped up in a victim mentality, then you're, at least partially, resigned to it as a matter of fact. If you have developed a negative thought model of your world, you will most likely continue to attract the same things into it. However, once you take full responsibility for everything in your life, including your thoughts, attitude and feelings, your life will begin to change. This may sound like a daunting task, but it's worth taking some moral inventory. Once you clear the mind, you can reach for a thought that produces a more pleasurable feeling.

One of the first things I do with my clients is have a conversation about personal responsibility. When you take responsibility for everything in your life past and present, it's a proclamation to the universe. Wayne Dyer said, "Change the way you look at things and the things that you look at will change." You cannot wait for things to change; you must become the change itself.

The next thing we do is get them moving and breathing. A more formal practice will help to steer their attention inward, into the body through breath. This will begin the process of disrupting and eventually dismantling thought patterns. This will also get the body on board into the feeling mode. When we're in touch with what we're thinking and feeling, we are on our way to healing.

When you breathe in almost any specific way, it takes your undivided attention to both feel and coordinate inhales, pauses and exhales. The more sophisticated breath-work, such as with Ujjayi Pranayama, the more attention it requires. You light up more parts of the brain, recruiting more muscles and nerves to receive feedback from more body parts. Instead of worrying about something in the past or the future, your concern becomes more immediate. Things that you normally worry about drift further away as you get pulled into the present moment of the next breath and body part. The more you move the breath and body in unison, the more sensation you receive and the more your thoughts become fleeting and distant.

As more time goes by the busy, dry erase board of your mind will be wiped clean. When you stop moving the breath and body, some time will pass by without any thoughts. A clear mind. Meditation. This is a great place to just enjoy being. At some point, thoughts will begin to flutter their way back in. A daily practice provides enough space for you to begin seeing and hearing what those thoughts, voices and commentary are saying and what you're feeling.

Thoughts and feelings are directly connected. Your feelings will give you an indication of your thoughts. As you uncover negative thoughts that create negative feelings, you can start to question them and question what thought would feel better.

When we keep ourselves moving in the direction of what feels good, naturally, it will help us move toward, or attract what we want. That doesn't mean that difficult things won't happen, and we'll never feel bad, we just don't allow ourselves to be taken over. It means that when things happen, we know we're not being singled out by the universe or punished. In addition, we make sure that we do not punish ourselves for causing the situation in the first place. Shit happens.

In 2007, I purchased a house at the height of the real estate market before the 2008 crash. I bought high. I didn't do my research and got caught up in the buying frenzy. Within a few months of owning my first house, I realized I was in over my head. I was barely able to make my mortgage payments. At the same time, I was struggling to keep my first yoga studio in operation. The next several months were brutal. First, my great uncle died. He was like a grandfather to me and a father to my mom. Then my grandmother died, whom I was very close with. She was the matriarch of the family. We visited her nearly every week from the time I was an infant. Then, my wolf dog, Codi, died a few weeks after that. He was a huge influence in my life. I had so many amazing experiences with him. We had even lived on a wolf refuge together in CO. Shortly after that, the yoga studio went belly up. Then, I defaulted on my mortgage. Then, the $30,000 loan I was supposed to receive from the bank for a new studio location, collapsed and I got nothing. I had already signed a five-year lease for the new studio space. I remember walking out of the bank. It was 105 degrees. I felt like I got punched in the face and the universe was conspiring against me. I questioned, if all the hard work I had put into my life was all for nothing. I felt defeated, yet I still somehow dragged myself into a Yoga practice every day to breathe, move and be still.

The story gets even better, or worse depending on how you look at it. I stayed true to my vision, which was to open a new Yoga studio. Self-defeating thoughts swirled around in my head, but I was aware of them, which gave me the mental fortitude to call "bullshit" on them and steer my actions forward toward my vision. Despite many people telling me that I shouldn't, I used credit cards to purchase everything I needed for the new studio and built the rest by hand. A close friend loaned me $5000, but it went fast. My girlfriend and I had moved into a tiny one-bedroom apartment. For months we skimmed by. In less than five years we separated and sold the business for $120,000, each getting $60,000.

I then co-founded a brand-new business called Take15Now. My business partner and I raised $100,000 from investors including family. We were sure that our new product was something that every business needed. Actually, it was, but you have to sell people on the great idea. We didn't know how to sell it, because it had never been done before. In less than two years, we were done. I lost it all. I was nearly suicidal after that. On top of my own financial ruin, I lost everyone else's money as well. The grief went deep. I blamed myself and it was unrelenting.

For most men, financial wealth is a reflection of our ability to provide security and is part of our masculinity and identity. With seemingly nothing left, I was triggered into a dark place. My internal dialogue was brutal. I fell back into a whiskey bottle for a time, but still fumbled my way onto the Yoga mat kicking and screaming. I breathed deeply and cried, moved and cried some more until I finally rested. It cleared my mind enough for me to embody the one thing that I knew was still true, the one thing that I clung to, the one thing that had been proven by people much smarter than me: I am, as you are, a living breathing miracle with an extreme intelligence coursing through every cell of our body. I was able to sit with the guilt and shame and self-talk and re-shape it. Yoga saved my life again, because I continued to participate in the truth of what I am. This is what I help people to embody within themselves.

1. Commit 100% to doing your own daily Yoga practice, a spiritual practice of breathing, moving and resting deeply, so that the mind can settle into and once again become the body itself. When this merging takes place again and again, you will begin to see more clearly. Adhering to a daily Yoga practice that follows the principles of practice outlined in the previous chapters is the single most empowering thing you can do for yourself, your family and the planet, period. If you make it a priority it will naturally weave its way into your day. After a while you won't feel like yourself unless you do your Yoga. That's where you want to be. If you do it regardless of any obstacles or excuses, whether you feel like it or not, you will feel supported by the universe.

Over time, you will notice and feel more with your body, because when the mind releases the constant regurgitation of repeated thought patterns it will reveal the goose with the golden eggs. You will begin to hear your own self-talk when in rest or meditation or out in the world. Knowing what you tell yourself or how you speak to yourself on a daily basis is to participate fully in your own reality.

2. Reprogram your attitude with the words that you speak. There are several scientific studies confirming the efficacy of affirmation, meaning your words have power. Whatever you tell yourself and others repetitively, the mind wants to make true. This can work for or against you.

Don Miguel Ruiz in his bestselling book, *The Four Agreements,* calls this particular agreement: *Be Impeccable with Your Word.* He shares this ancient toltec wisdom from his ancestry that has withstood the test of time. It's a known fact that the words you recite on a regular basis have power, so choose them deliberately.

A mantra is a word or phrase repeated over and over to help the mind concentrate. Herbert Benson proved that using mantra in meditation elicits the Relaxation Response.[11] So if you're repeating something that you don't want to be true, flush it out, stop it and replace it with a new phrase that empowers and directs.

Your new practices will help you to become more mindful and aware of what words you're thinking and literally speaking. If you say: "I am tired, I am stuck, I am struggling, I am having a hard time, I am anxious,

---

[11] Benson, Herbert, M.D., Relaxation Response, 2001

I am stressed…over and over the mind will do its best to grant you that wish, because that's how the mind works. This is neuroscience. Most of these speech patterns are well established. Your job is to become aware of them, then interrupt these patterns by consciously changing them. Most people speak with little awareness as to what they're actually expressing to other people beyond their words. The body has its own language, and it may or may not be aligned with the words coming out of someone's mouth. The sound, tone, speed and posture reveals its own story.

Personally, I am fascinated by what people say and how they say it while in conversation. This has become a large part of my work. It's called active listening. It's a critical skill that I've developed over the years. When we listen with our full attention and physical presence, we pick up on subtle or even blatant nuances. We might notice when someone is sabotaging themselves. For instance, if someone wants less stress in their life, yet they keep telling their friends how stressed they are all the time, they're misaligned.

A great exercise in cultivating better listening skills is to listen with your whole body and being when you're in a conversation with someone. Dial into them. Not just with your ears, but with your full presence and senses. Notice their body language. Does what they're saying feel true? What words are they using? What are you hearing beyond their words? This is active listening. Pay especially close attention when someone begins a sentence with "I", "I am", or "I'm the type of person who…." Take notice of what they're saying about themselves and listen to how you feel when they're talking. As you practice these listening skills, you'll begin to notice more and more the words and sentiments that you also use. The better you are at listening to others, the better you'll get at listening to what you say when you speak. Whenever you can catch yourself saying something that's not true or that you don't want to be true, or when you're being more negative than you want to be, it's an opportunity to rewrite your story.

When I catch myself saying something that has a negative connotation or that simply isn't true, I'll take a minute and say it over in a new way, an empowered way. I do this in conversation or even when I'm alone. I call this "communication clean up". In order to recalibrate a healthier mindset, we have to clean up what we say and how we say it, so that we can generate the truth from a positive empowered place within us. If this place doesn't already exist within us, we must create it, declare it. If we say something enough, we'll believe it and live it out despite it not even being true. Especially things that we repeat often that disempowers us. Most likely you have "go-to" phrases that are automatic responses. What are these? "I am always tired. I'm really busy. I'm fine. I am not a morning person. I hate my job. I have anxiety. My anxiety does this or that...I have no time. Same old, same old. I'm bored. You make me feel...."

One of my clients kept repeating the phrase: "I have so much anxiety all the time." "I have so much anxiety all the time." "I have so much anxiety...." She didn't realize how much she said it on a regular basis. If you say something enough, you'll believe it even if it's not true. It becomes a self-fulfilling prophecy. I am not implying that she didn't have anxiety, but she kept reinforcing it with a disempowering mantra. We immediately reshaped that phrase into, "I am feeling better and better in my body."

This was the phrase that resonated most with her, but it can be almost anything with a positive spin. We implemented her new mantra in two ways. Whenever her friends or family asked her how she was doing her reply would be: "I am feeling better and better in my body." In addition, she wrote her new phrase in her journal 20 times per day for 20 days immediately following her Yoga practice, when her mind was clear and she was connected to her body. It didn't take long for her to turn a corner. She literally felt better and better in her body. It's not that her anxiety was gone forever, but she was better able to call bullshit on her own words and the thought patterns that created it. Her Yoga practice grounds her in reality and the truth of her body, so she can actualize whatever is happening in her life and integrate positive thought patterns.

Positive statements or affirmations alone are not very useful, but when you couple them with a physical and spiritual practice, you re-write your script. When you catch yourself saying something that is negative or disempowering and replace it with a statement that has a positive charge, while being connected to your body, you're reprogramming the mind. You're no longer on autopilot, you're mindfully choosing your words and therefore reworking thoughts. When you say the new positive statement, take notice of how you feel when you say it. Take a deep breath, place one hand on your heart and hold one hand up in the air like you're taking an oath. Eventually, if you stay the course, disempowering words won't even come out of your mouth. Positive affirmations by themselves have limited power, but let's not forget that you are also tilling the soil of your new garden, your body. You're learning to trust the body's wisdom and intelligence. A great time to reinforce healthy communication is just after your Yoga practice. If you really take this on, your friends will notice something different about you. You'll be living more in the present moment; awake, alive and appreciating your miracle.

I have put some journaling exercises at the end of this chapter to do daily. I suggest doing the writing exercise in the morning after your Yoga practice to establish a healthy rapport as you move into your day. In essence, you are training yourself to be more loving and intentional with the words you speak both to yourself and others.

Negative self-talk likely took years to develop in you, therefore the first step is to understand that you are in a process and practice of patience, kindness, and compassion. You're allowing your Yoga: breathwork, movement, meditation, and your own unique nature to ground you. You are becoming more intimate with your body and life. Keep the faith! As one of my first teachers, the late Michael Hopp instilled in me:

"Just keep putting in the good and whatever doesn't belong will eventually fall away."

While you're becoming more mindful and putting in the good, you'll naturally gravitate toward what feels good and pleases you. Follow that stream of feel good. A hot bath, a steam, a pedicure, a massage, a movie, a workout, a walk in nature, coffee with a friend. These will support you loving yourself. Do the things that feel good and keep you connected to your body as much as possible, so you're feeding the positive. If you're not use to caring for yourself in this way, guilt may show up. I've heard people say: "I feel like I'm being selfish." You might believe that you don't deserve to feel good, but that is a lie that many people tell themselves. We are re-establishing your self-worth. Guilt has a voice, what is it? Get clear about what you're saying to yourself and what you actually believe around this that is not true. Get to the truth. When you uncover a word or phrase that sabotages you, ask yourself: Is it true?

Here's the truth: You are a miracle! Caring for your miracle is never ever wrong or bad. When you nurture your miracle of life all the other important relationships in your life will also blossom.

The combination of clarity, satisfaction, and intention is an indomitable force of nature, because together they help you navigate forward empowered and confident. While you build this new level of awareness into your daily life you will become more proficient at communicating to the self, other people, and the universe. As outlined in previous chapters we communicate to the self by our actions and thoughts. Your Yoga practice all by itself communicates alignment, love, and safety by participating in the reality of your breath and body. This intimate connection allows you to feel more. Your feelings in the present will give you a roadmap to your future. Your words matter. The combination of feeling more, feeling good, and using words that are positive and intentional will pave the way forward and lift your spirits in a genuinely powerful way.

<u>Daily Writing Exercise:</u>

If you want to be a positive person, if you want to shift anxiety and stress into empowerment and freedom, you must reprogram your language and thoughts around your words.

1. Do Your Yoga: breathe, move, meditate, write to yourself!

2. What do you say and how do you say it? Notice what negative things you say often. Write these things out on paper, so you can get a look at them, materialize them outside of your brain and body. Pull them out of you, so you can begin the process of recalibrating.

3. Re-write the script. Create new go to statements that oppose your negative ones but are honest and truthful. Write three positive statements about yourself, a commitment, the work you're doing, or the direction you want to go. This will help you harness the power of intention and positive thinking. Write the statements out 20 times for each one and say them aloud 10-20 times per day. Use I Am…statements. Be bold. This may feel awkward at first. Do it anyway.

Ex. I Am a miracle! I Am empowered and confident! I Am disciplined, positive and courageous in all of my endeavors! I am in a process of discovering new wonders about myself.

Remember, positive affirmations only work when you have a genuine connection to your heart and body. Do your Yoga first and you will be more open to receive the affirmations.

Chapter 13
<u>Detox Your Body, Feed Your Soul</u>

The foods you eat have a direct effect on your mental health. There's plenty of research indicating that a well-balanced, nutrient rich diet that is low in saturated fats and sugars and high in plant content supports mental health. It seems probable that there might be as many studies as there are diet books on healthy eating and cooking, so I will cut to the chase: eat as clean as possible.

In the following chapter, I introduce eight principles for cleaning up everything around eating. In addition, you'll find a four-day detox at the end of this chapter. Our objectives here are to: 1. detox your digestive system and organs, 2. establish a healthy relationship with food.

When I say eat clean, I mean eat foods close to the source from which they came. Stay away from too many chemicals, pesticides and GMO's. In fact, do your best to eat organic if possible. When buying packaged foods, look for short ingredient lists that are not laden with manmade artificial chemicals and preservatives created in a lab. Take full responsibility for what goes into your precious miracle body.

The idea is to keep the digestive system running as clean and as efficiently as possible. There are several detox formulas and products on the market that offer ways to promote a healthy gut. Some are more radical than others. I only use products that I have researched and verified in terms of their safety and what they accomplish. I suggest beginning with a simple four-day cleanse to start, so you can see how your body reacts. At the end of this chapter, you'll find a safe, gentle, proven way to clean out and stimulate organ function with no harsh side effects whatsoever. It will go along perfectly with your Yoga practice. As you clean up what goes into your miraculous body, I recommend taking a look at your behaviors around eating.

You may not think about eating as a way of communicating, but that's exactly what it is. The food you eat conveys a message to your body and being. Good nutrition and healthy eating habits send love and healing to your inner being. It's literally informing your body on a cellular and energetic level. You cannot expect to move the needle on anxiety if your diet is thwarting your efforts. Consuming large amounts of sugar, fried food and saturated fats are linked to higher rates of inflammation in the body and a decreased number of good bacteria. When you consume fresh, nutrient rich foods that are closer to the source from which they came, you can literally taste and feel the difference.

Every year my dad and I grow a garden. There's no comparison to eating vibrant, phytonutrient rich vegetables plucked from the plant it grew on. Recent studies have proven that a healthy gut biome positively influences everything from our immune system to the thoughts we think.

Your digestive system processes more than just food, it's also tied directly to your emotions. Stress and anxiety effects digestion, and digestion can alter one's mood. In fact, the intestines are the main production center of serotonin, an important neurotransmitter that helps stabilize our mood. We all have to process what we take in through our senses and when stressed or anxious, our body first works to secure our safety. If we are chronically functioning in the flight or fight response, the digestive system itself may partially shut down depending on the level of fear we're living with. Many people who are knowingly or unknowingly stressed, have digestive issues. Stress affects the digestive system's ability to breakdown and extract the nutrients from food. As you know, the opposite of the stress response is the rest and digest or Relaxation Response. When you're relaxed and grounded, your digestive system works most efficiently. For this reason, the first meal that you eat after your Yoga practice is especially important, because you'll be in a restful space and your body will be ready to receive and absorb.

The idea here, is to feed yourself the essentials and cut out all the extras, so that your body can function optimally. You and only you ultimately have control over what you consume. When you upgrade your mindset and make choices that feed your soul, rather than your emotions and pleasure centers, you communicate safety, control, self-love, and clarity. The principles below are a guide to help you do exactly that. They are not rules. Follow all of them and you will experience a major shift. Follow any of them and shift will happen proportionately.

<u>Body Wisdom Training Nutritional Principles</u>

1. Eat for fuel only.
2. Eat only clean food, avoid processed foods.

3. Drink more water (women approx. 2.75 liters and men approx. one gallon).
4. Supplement key vitamins and minerals. (Appendix B)
5. Avoid: fried foods, white sugar, large quantities of alcohol, GMO's - especially corn, wheat, or soy.
6. Detox and get empty periodically.
7. Probiotics, fermentation and a healthy gut.
8. The "first thing in", principle.

<u>1. Eat For Fuel Only</u>

Why are you eating? Interestingly enough, why you eat is as important as what you eat. Are you eating because you're actually hungry or you're emotional? Are you feeling lonely, sad, angry, shame? Are you bored? Are you stuffing your face to numb out? Most of us get an urge to eat when we are not actually hungry. When we eat with our emotions it almost always makes us feel worse. Not only are the feelings of why you ate a half gallon of ice cream or an entire bag of potato chips still lingering, but guilt might then be thrown in on top. When you eat for fuel only, you are streamlining the reason to eat at all. To fuel and feed your mind, body and soul only. Whatever your body doesn't need and doesn't burn up will either be excreted or stored.

Before you put anything in your mouth, stop, take a breath and ask yourself: is what I'm about to eat for fuel or something else? In other words, is the thing that you're about to eat supplying you with nutrition or is it sabotaging you in some way? If it's the later, the next question is: why am I eating this? It's a very straightforward question and at the very least will help you become more mindful no matter what the answer is and no matter what you decide to do. If the answer is clearly that you're about to emotionally eat, take action! Pull out your notebook or journal and write down what you're feeling and why. Are you angry? Lonely? Disappointed? Sad? Write it out. Get it out of you. Even if you still decide to eat that thing, you'll see more clearly the emotional connection to eating. This principle alone has a great power to disrupt and break your habitual eating patterns and help you uncover the truth. I have clients that have lost a significant amount of weight using this one principle.

2. Eat Only Clean Food, Avoid Highly Processed Foods

What are you eating? I'm not going to go into a long dissertation about the food supply in the United States. What I can tell you is our food supply chain and sources of food are suspect. The majority of big food companies from growers to manufacturers to distributors are corporate entities, which for the most part means profit over everything else including you. Corporate farms use Genetically Modified Organisms (GMO's), which means the seeds have been engineered to function in a certain way. These foods are not allowed as a food source to humans in over 60 countries around the world including Italy, Germany, France, Greece, and Venezuela to name a few. In many nations GMO's must be labeled, but not in the U.S. In fact, many conventional fruits and veggies are laden with things that, given the choice, I personally try to avoid. Things like glyphosate, petroleum, fertilizers, chemical enhancers, and other strange ways to bring foods to market faster and make them look good.

Food stored on the shelves of supermarkets contain many things to enhance, preserve and entice you, including their packaging. Some of those foods might be approved by the FDA but are still nutritionally debatable. When a product has an extensive ingredient list, I generally stay away from it. The longer the list, the more likely it has crap in it. When you eat that shit, your body may not know what to do with it or how to process it. If you trust the source, then it's up to you, but I have done enough of my own research to be skeptical. I don't want my body to have to work extra hard to sort out and deal with all those chemicals. If your body can't use the materials that are put into it, it may not know what to do with them. If it doesn't burn them up, it will either store them or try to excrete them if it can. Some things have an accumulative affect in the body and will damage your cells over time, such as glyphosate. This is another reason we want to turn up the metabolic flame to burn through or excrete what doesn't belong. Your daily Yoga practice and your food choices will help you to do exactly that.

3. Drink Enough Water

There's plenty of research out there proving the benefits of staying hydrated. Not only does it keep organs flushed, especially your kidneys that filter waste from your blood, but also lowers your risk of anxiety and depression. [12] The recommended daily amount of water for women is approximately 2.5 quartz and for men, just under one gallon. That may seem like a lot, but everything you drink is added together, even coffee and tea. Although, coffee and caffeinated tea are a diuretic, they do not necessarily dehydrate you unless you're not drinking enough other fluids. The main idea here is that you hydrate throughout the day. The body is around 60% water, so it's not rocket science to understand how important it is. Personally, I fill a jug of water and drink off of it all day long. That way I can measure my intake. Also, water aids in digestion across the board. I've heard some people complain that when they drink a lot, they also need to go to the bathroom a lot. Yes! This keeps the system flushed, muscles and joints lubricated, and cells hydrated. In fact, the first thing the doctor tells us when we get sick is to stay hydrated.

4. Supplement Key Vitamins, Minerals and Nutrients Daily

Your body is made up of a vast network of materials and tissues that are building and repairing constantly. In order for your brain and body to function optimally it needs certain key nutrients. In fact, a growing number of nutritional experts believe that many ailments and issues will literally disappear if the body gets what it needs. A diet high in saturated fats, sugar and refined carbohydrates is not heart healthy and

---

[12] Haghighatdoost F, Feizi A, Esmaillzadeh A, Rashidi-Pourfard N, Keshteli AH, Roohafza H, Adibi P., 2018

likely not good for your head either. The combination of taking in too much bad stuff and being deficient in the good stuff can impact the chemistry of your mind and body. If your body doesn't get what it needs, it will not be able to sufficiently carryout the millions of chemical reactions that it must perform on a daily basis. If we're taking full responsibility for everything in our lives, getting enough nutrients should be at the top of the list.

If the majority of your calories come from plant material and you eat a variety of foods, a good multi-vitamin might be enough for you. I take a wide range of supplements to make sure my body is getting everything it needs, especially my brain.

The average American diet is deficient in some key nutrients such as: vitamin A, B6, C & D, iron, calcium, potassium, and magnesium to name a few. It's not just from not eating healthy, it's also from soil depletion. The soils across America's farmlands have been stripped and depleted from key nutrients not being replenished over the last 50 years.

<u>Here's a short list of key nutrients:</u>
Vitamin B's full spectrum, Vitamins: C, D, E, K, Magnesium, Iron, Zinc, Omega 3's (Refer to Appendix B for a complete list.)

<u>5. Avoid fried foods, white sugar, artificial sweeteners, refined carbs, low quality dairy, large quantities of alcohol and GMO's.</u>

- Fried foods wreak havoc on your gut bacteria and cause inflammation. Healthy gut bacteria are important for digestion, immune system function and overall health. The majority of oil used in commercial fryers is highly refined and often oxidized or burnt. I've been to many restaurants across the country that have served food cooked in burnt oil. Saturated fats and oils that have been broken down over time by high heat is basically like eating a plate full of poison in my opinion. That's no exaggeration.

- White refined sugar is also toxic. It's a major contributor of diabetes, obesity, high blood pressure, heart disease, anxiety and depression.

- There are conflicting scientific reports about whether or not artificial sweeteners, such as the ones in diet soda, are bad for you. Anything that says artificial, I stay away from. These sweeteners are labeled as food additives by the FDA. Real food doesn't need additives.

- Refined carbs are basically grains that have been stripped of their fiber, bran, and many of their nutrients. These include things like candy, white breads, pastries, many commercial brands of breakfast cereals, etc.

- Many commercial dairy products contain growth hormone and antibiotics given to the cows that produce it. American cheeses are pasteurized, which makes them different then many European cheeses that are aged naturally. If you buy imported cheese from Italy that has been aged naturally, it will generally have a better quality. I am personally lactose intolerant, so I can only eat sheep or goat cheese. Humans are the only adult mammals that drink milk. If we're getting enough protein and calcium, we don't necessarily need milk in our diet at all. If you love cheese, go for naturally aged, high-quality cheese.

- GMO: Genetically Modified Organism. One of the biggest concerns about GMO's is that many are sprayed with herbicides some containing glyphosate, which has been proven to cause cancer. In fact, there's currently a huge class action case involving the herbicide Round Up, which was originally manufactured by Monsanto, the largest seed producer in the world. Over 100,000 people have sued them so far, with settlements reaching into the billions. According to the Environmental Protection Agency, in the U.S. "About 280 million pounds of glyphosate are applied to 298 million acres annually."[13] The herbicide is used in soy, corn, wheat and other mass-produced crops, so do your best to avoid conventional brands. Buy either non-GMO brands or organic.

---

[13] Caleb Hawkins, Environmental Protection Agency, Memorandum, April 2018

6. <u>The Importance of Getting Empty</u>

While this isn't for everyone, getting empty is helpful for metabolism and the body's ability to clean out. Of course, I recommend consulting with your doctor before drastically changing your eating habits. When we allow ourselves to go for 12-15 hours without food it gives our digestive tract a break. We don't need to keep the stomach constantly full during our waking hours. In fact, there's a lot to be said for what has become known as intermittent fasting. Basically, you have your biggest meal of the day in the early afternoon and a small meal in the evening. If you don't consume anything else, besides water or tea, you will allow your body a nice digestive rest. During that time your body is cleaning and doing maintenance. Not only that, but those who subscribe to intermittent fasting swear that it increases metabolism to burn excess fat and anything else that might need removal. I am on board for sure!

7. <u>The "First Thing In" Principle</u>

What is the first thing that you put in your body every day? This principle seems logical to me especially if you've allowed yourself to be empty for 12 hours. It asks you to be mindful of the first thing that you put into your body. It can even go beyond eating, like making sure the first thing that you read or listen to are positive and supportive.

When it comes to eating or drinking, do your best to make the first thing in as healthy as you can. Most mornings I take a charcoal capsule with a full 16oz. glass of water. On the days that I don't take charcoal, I drink a full glass of warm lemon water. The first food source I take in is organic micro green powder with probiotic mixed with coconut milk. Sometimes I'll add a mushroom complex powder for good measure. This mixture is loaded with phytonutrients. In addition to the "first thing in" principle for nutrition, what is the first thing that you say to yourself when you wake up? Before I even get out of bed in the morning, I cite a gratitude list in my mind with one hand on my heart and the other on my belly. The "first thing in" principle helps you to start your day off with a win.

8. <u>Fermentation and Probiotics For Gut Health</u>

The importance of a healthy bacterial biome in the stomach and intestines cannot be overstated. There is tons of evidence confirming that healthy gut bacteria reduces inflammation, increases immune system response, supports the cardiovascular system, brain chemistry and overall health of the body. You could simply eat or drink fermented foods regularly such as: kombucha, sauerkraut, miso, kimchi, naturally aged cheeses, plain yogurt and kefir. Even wine, beer or cider can be healthy sources of good bacteria, depending on quality and quantity.

I'm always a fan of nature providing what we need. However, if you don't consume fermented foods regularly probiotics are a wise choice. They will add healthy bacteria to your intestinal tract.

A quick note on coffee. There's some controversy about coffee and whether or not it's good for you. Recent studies lean toward coffee being good for you, but it depends on many other factors. I am not going to take a stand one way or the other. I will say, if you drink coffee, go organic and use brown paper filters to brew it. For most people with anxiety, stress and overthinking, it's recommended that you steer clear of caffeine in general, including coffee.

Detoxification, Cleaning Out The Digestive System

While there might be conflicting information about whether or not detoxing the digestive system is necessary, in my experience I always feel better when I do. I have more energy and less brain fog. I tend to lean into a more holistic approach to health, such as the ancient medical system of Ayurveda. Ayurveda is about using diet and other practices to keep the body in a harmonious, balanced state. One of the ways is by turning up the heat of digestion. Cleaning out our digestive system and stimulating organ function can be of great benefit. Not only is a detox healthy for your body, but also continues to build rapport between the mind/body/spirit relationship.

A detox might sound uncomfortable, even dreadful, especially if you associate it with cleaning out your colon to prepare for a colonoscopy. That's not what I'm talking about here. I'm referring to a much gentler, user friendly approach to internal cleansing. Regardless, if thoughts about a cleanse are going to ramp up your anxiety, do it with someone qualified to support you through it.

The body works, in part, like a filtration system. We have to filter all kinds of debris coming into the body through the air we breathe and food we eat. You might think of a detox in the body like cleaning your filters. When we replace or clean out the filter in our vacuum or furnace it runs more efficiently. Otherwise, the filter gets clogged and the appliance has to work harder than necessary. When you do a cleanse, you will most definitely notice a difference. After a detox people report having more energy, better bowel movements, a feeling of lightness, clarity, and mental sharpness.

If you haven't ever done any kind of cleanse, then start small. There are many types of cleanses out there, some are quite intense such as The Master Cleanse. This involves consuming nothing but, a solution of: lemon water, grade B maple syrup and cayenne pepper in the right proportion for consecutive days. People swear by it, but it's quite intense and perhaps unnecessary. A simple water fast is also a great way to clean out. Drink only water for a few days. There's plenty of products on the market that do the work for you. They contain herbs and plant materials that naturally stimulate and clean internal organs. Flor-Essence is one that I highly recommend. The ingredients are certified organic with a full spectrum of wonderful herbs designed and proven to clean the organs. In my online program, I take participants through a four-day detox. Below is the simple version of it.

<u>A Four Day Detox.</u>

*If you have a medical condition, consult with your doctor prior to altering your diet, especially if you're on medication or are diabetic.

Here's my suggestion for a four-day cleanse. Eat light for these four consecutive days. I'm not suggesting you starve yourself or suffer in any way. You can take the following recommendation and apply it as you see fit. Refer to Appendix B for a list of the supplements to use for the detox.

Begin your days with one charcoal capsule and a full glass of water 12-16 oz. at room temperature. Drink another glass of room temperature water within the hour. This will start you out well hydrated. You can work your way up to two capsules of charcoal by day three or four if it agrees with your system. Constipation is a sign that you need to back off the charcoal and drink more water. Medications and vitamins should be taken at least an hour prior to or after consuming charcoal.

After at least 90 minutes from taking your charcoal, drink the Flor-Essence Herbal Tea. Drink it slowly, mindfully, and as you do, perhaps say to yourself, 'I love my body, mind, and spirit.' Flor-Essence is packed with herbs and minerals that cleanse and stimulate organ function, including your digestive tract, kidneys, and liver. It acts as a tonic, it's gentle, yet a highly effective daily detox that is held in high regard.

Eat your first meal 15-30 minutes after you drink the tea. Make your first meal light and nutritious. Eat as clean as possible.

Here are some examples of a healthy first meal:
1. Carrot juice w/ whole grain toast and almond butter.
2. A cup of blueberries and or a banana with Tea or your favorite beverage

3.   A smoothie with frozen berries, banana, micro green powder

4.   Bowl of oatmeal w/ nut butter or walnuts.

5.   Eggs and whole grain bread.

6.   Your favorite organic cereal with berries and nuts.

*Remember: eat organic or at least non-GMO whenever possible.

When you feel empty again in an hour or so, take your psyllium husk powder mixed with water.

*Note: Once you put the powder into the water, mix it quickly and drink immediately. Make sure you drink the recommended amount of water daily.

Wait an hour or so, then have your one big healthy meal of the day with any additional supplements that you want to take (Appendix B). During the hour before your meal is a great time to do your Yoga practice.

Your main meal should be high on veggies and low on starchy carbs, such as breads and pastas. Broccoli, carrots, and cauliflower with fish is a great meal. Wild caught or organic raised salmon is best. Sardines is another, because they provide good fats and protein. I understand that many people don't like sardines, but you can go with organic chicken or lean organic grass-fed beef if you eat meat. If you're a vegetarian or vegan go with good organic tofu or tempeh. A small helping of rice is fine but make the bulk of the meal vegetables. Avocados are excellent. Any leafy green vegetable is good as well. Try to include colorful veggies throughout your cleanse and beyond: reds, greens, blues, yellows etc. Peppers, kale, carrots, cauliflower, tomatoes, etc. Colors in fruits and veggies contain antioxidants that help to protect your cells from damage.

By mid-day or early evening have another cup of the Flor-Essence Tea.

Some people won't need any more food, but if you do, have another small meal. It could be hummus with carrot and celery sticks. Or make yourself a salad with dark green leafy lettuce like mescaline greens or spinach or baby kale with your favorite nuts.

Take notice that you're eating to appreciate your amazing body and mind. Eat as much organic fruit as you want in-between your meals, but keep in mind that most fruit has a high sugar content. Try to be done eating by 7 or 8pm at the latest.

Drink your third cup of Flor-Essence Tea an hour or so after your last meal.

Avoid overeating. Eat mindfully. Breathe between bites. Enjoy the food that is providing you with sustenance, nourishment and clean energy. If thoughts or emotions come up while cleansing, journal about them. What are you feeling? Thinking? What narratives or stories surface while you're eating clean and mindfully?

Hopefully, the four-day cleanse will inspire you to eat healthier in general. You could extend it to seven days. I eat like this normally. I take charcoal about three times per week first thing in the morning and psyllium husk w/ probiotic shortly thereafter. The majority of my diet is plant based. Flor-Essence is something I take for about two weeks, four times per year.

Nutritional Tropical Blend:

One of my favorite things to eat while on a cleanse or anytime the produce is fresh is a tropical blend of papaya, mango, and avocado. These are delicious and nutritious together. You get good fats and proteins from the avocados, while mangos and papaya together provide excellent vitamins, minerals and enzymes. In the Summer when it's hot out, I might eat this blend for every meal for consecutive days in a row.

Preparation: You'll need: one medium to large papaya (use half), 3 or 4 avocados, and 3 or 4 mangos. I like using yellow honey or champagne mangos. First, wash all produce. Peel the fruit. Cut into cubes and add equal parts of each fruit in a large bowl. Squeeze fresh lime juice over the top, salt to taste, stir gently and enjoy! If you like spice, add some cayenne pepper.

I have experimented with several cleanses and detoxes through the years, and some are more intense than others. You have to find the right one for you. The Body Wisdom Nutritional Principles will help you shift into a new perspective and cleaner diet overall. I am 100% confident that being more conscious of what you consume will support everything that you do in life.

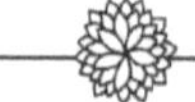

Chapter 14
Hot and Cold Therapy

As a wrestler in high school, sweating profusely was part of my daily routine. Besides the grueling practices we would often jump rope in the boiler room with plastic suits on to sweat out a few pounds. The rationale was purely strategic. Wrestling at the lightest weight possible gave us an edge over our opponent. Soon enough we were introduced to the dry sauna and steam room. It was less work than jumping rope and it became more therapeutic. As long as I didn't overdo it and stayed hydrated, I always felt great after a good sweat.

The skin is the largest organ in the body and has a great capacity to detox and purify the system through sweating. It was designed this way. Not only that, but when you're sitting in a room that is 120 degrees or more, you get present quickly. Many cultures around the world have used heat therapy to induce sweat for purification purposes. I first began attending sweat lodge ceremonies during massage school in the mid 90's. It wasn't until I sat on the ground in a traditional Lakota Sweat Lodge listening to prayer songs, did I have some kind of spiritual awakening. I was told that the steam from the water poured on the rocks is the breath of Mother Earth. It sure felt like that. When the only door, which was made from a thick canvas, was closed the temperature soared and it was pitch dark except from the glow of the lava rocks. All I could do was focus on my breath and feel the beat of the drum and listen to voice of the singers. Not only was I sweating out toxins, but praying with my whole heart, body and soul. I have been sweating regularly in various ways for over 30 years. I am a firm believer in both exercise induced sweat and overheating the body in a restful state. The benefits far outweigh the uncomfortableness, but it's not for everyone. Nothing is. You must find what works for you.

If you choose to sweat regularly, it's paramount that you replenish key vitamins and minerals, such as vit. C, potassium, magnesium and selenium to name a few. If you're new to sweating in a heated environment, begin slow and build up your tolerance over time. Your body and mind will adapt. It's this adaptive ability or neural plasticity and flexibility that we're after. Many benefits will follow, including overall purification by flushing toxins out, disease prevention, increased efficiency in temperature control, healthier skin and pores, increase in endorphins and metabolic rate.

Hot tubs are another place to overheat the body. In a hot tub, you may not even know you're sweating, so remember to stay hydrated and time yourself. If you're new to using heat, chances are you do not yet have the sensitivity and ability to know when enough is enough. Set a timer. Safety is most important. **Avoid** drinking alcohol when using heat therapy. It will dehydrate you quickly.

If you don't have access to a place to sweat, such as a gym or recreation center, you can create a steam room in your bathroom with a hot shower. Or be creative and figure out a way to break a sweat a few times per week. Just make sure it's safe!

Cold Therapy

When I was 25, I went fishing from the shore of Blue Mesa Reservoir in Gunnison, Colorado. It was Spring and the sun was out, but the wind was brisk. The water was frigid from snow melt. I don't know what came over me, but I decided to jump in the lake. The water was so cold, it took my breath away. My chest constricted and I began to panic. A guy standing on shore yelled to me: "just breathe slow and deep." So, I did and was able to regain control of my breath. I tread water only for a few minutes before I climbed out. As soon as I did, I noticed hang gliders in the distance playing in the wind above the mountainside. I felt amazing! My mind was crystal clear, and my body felt light and clean. I was not cold at first, despite having goose bumps, I was stimulated. From that point forward while I was on the road, I jumped in every cold river, lake or pond that I could find. I was hooked. I have been using cold showers, plunges and ice baths ever since.

When I worked as a Massage Therapist at the Canyon Ranch in Tucson, Arizona, I would do several treatments back-to-back. My hands and forearms were pumped with blood and my joints became stiff. Each night before I left, I used the cold plunge to clear the inflammation out quickly. When I didn't have access to a full body cold plunge, I soaked my arms and hands in a five-gallon bucket of ice water. I swear by the benefits of cold therapy, and it has kept my arms, hands and fingers healthy after 25 years of massage therapy.

Low and behold, since my days of cold plunging on the road, Mr. Wim Hoff has defied the laws of nature and made ice baths a global phenomenon. To be fair cold therapy has been used by different cultures for hundreds, if not thousands of years. Today, cold therapy, specifically ice baths, are said to be like a miracle drug. Ice bath enthusiasts say that it strengthens blood vessels, stimulates the immune system, reduces or even wipes out inflammation, and wards off depression and anxiety, which is why I have included cold therapy in this book. The main reason they're helpful for mental health is because you must focus on breathing.

The thought of submerging yourself in ice cold water scares the crap out of most people. First of all, I do not suggest shocking yourself like I did. I was young and naive when I jumped in that water. Instead, train yourself gradually over time if you're curious. The first step is to use the right breathwork technique to charge the system. In Appendix A under the Seven Sacred Breaths, you'll find the **Cold Therapy Prep Breath**. This is the breathing technique to use before you enter cold therapy or water. Once you enter, remain calm, focused and maintain a slow, steady controlled breath.

You can start out by ending your normal shower with 30 seconds of cold water. Gradually turn the shower water to cold until you notice your body reacting by producing goose bumps. Control your breathing with slow steady breaths for at least 20 seconds. Let the cold water run on all sides of your body, then turn the water off. Do it again in your next shower. Make it a habit. You don't have to be obsessive about it but give it a try. Over the next week or two increase the duration and decrease the temperature until you're able to stay in for up to two to three minutes. Anywhere between 30 seconds and three minutes has great benefits. The temperature of the water coming out of your shower head will vary depending on where you live and what time of year it is. If you live in Florida or Arizona, it will most likely not be cold enough, but if you live in Chicago, it probably will.

If you choose to take it a step further and make it colder. An ice bath is the pinnacle of cold-water therapy.

*It is highly recommended that you train with a qualified coach.

Make sure you train yourself for a solid month with cold showers before you even attempt an ice bath. Even with ice baths, you'll want to gradually increase the cold.

Here's how I do it. I fill my tub with cold water. If it's winter in NY, that's cold enough for me. If I want it colder, I add ice or snow when available. Let's say a standard bag of ice is 5 lbs. I use about half a bag of ice with cold water. Over time, you can work your way up to a full bag or more. Honestly, the colder the better. It will do the work faster. Dr. Susanna Soeberg is a metabolic expert, and she says, 11 minutes per week in an ice bath works wonders. Per week! Not in one session! You don't necessarily even have to be that extreme. If you never go beyond remaining calm and in control of your breath for a 30 second cold shower, you will still reap great benefits for mental and physical health.

I never enjoy the moments before entering into cold water, because like many people, I hate being cold. However, I love the feeling afterwards. I love practicing mind over matter. I love having to focus my mind on breathing and remaining calm while being uncomfortable. Its empowering. It says that I, like you, can do whatever we focus our mind on. Of course, people have taken this to the extreme and get carried away with the challenge of it, but just explore it, play with it, make it your own. Remember, anxiety and stress is fear based and you're learning to trust your body's wisdom and intelligence. You're becoming a spiritual warrior. This kind of training is remarkably potent for all people, but especially for anyone wanting to alleviate mental disturbances and anxiety.

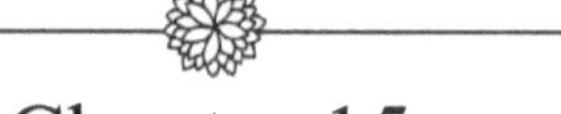

Chapter 15
<u>Sangha: Real Social Interaction and Community</u>

We need each other. Human beings are social creatures. We need to feel a sense of belonging. Too much time alone with our thoughts and feelings is detrimental to our self-preservation. We are meant to be part of an interactive community and must find ways and places to be socially accepted, connected, and appreciated.

Most indigenous cultures have a rite of passage for adolescent boys and girls when they are initiated into adulthood. They participate in ceremonies that empower them to have a voice in their community. It's often both a physical and spiritual ritual or endeavor. The Lakota have the vision quest and the Sun Dance ceremony. The community comes together in prayer, song, and dance to support those taking part. These ceremonies are centered around purification, healing, sacrifice and sending prayers to God or creator.

Many countries and cultures have their own rites of passage. In Thailand, it's common for boys to spend time with Buddhist monks or even become a monk for a time before they get married. In Jewish communities they have the Bar Mitzvah. In Japan they have what's called Seijin-no-Hi or "coming of age festival." The Latin community celebrates the Quinceanera, when girls enter womanhood at age 15. These gatherings honor and validate each individual as a vital part of the greater community.

While we see some traditions in America, there is no national rite of passage. Many people slip through the cracks of society, alone, as if they don't matter. This is especially detrimental to our youth. Teenagers look forward to their big day when they get their driver's license. When you turn 18 you can register to vote in public elections, but I wonder if we need something with a deeper community connection and meaning in our culture? Something more inclusive. A rite of passage that has more to do with giving something, rather than getting something. In a culture that puts so much emphasis on succeeding, we desperately need community integration. Perhaps, making things worse is social media that has artificially substituted the need for interaction with images on a screen. The truth is, people are starving for attention no matter how many "likes" they get. This has amplified the need for approval with superficial "likes," but nothing can replace someone's presence.

When we are alone for too long with an overactive mind and constant worry, it can be like a pressure cooker. The barrage of thoughts and inner dialogue builds in the brain and body. It's like the emoji of our head blowing up. It's not healthy for individuals or our greater society. This is how people felt during the pandemic with minimal real social interactions.

Mental health depends on our social habits, especially being heard and felt by someone else in real time. Otherwise, it's too easy to obsess and overthink everything, because it stays contained within. When someone is really listening to us, we feel validated.

When they nod and respond to us, we feel better, we feel a sense of being understood. We don't necessarily have to arrive at a solution about anything, just being heard can be enough. We all need people and places that we can share safely and openly what's really going on with us.

My dad has an expression that he uses when he doesn't think I'm listening, or he has to repeat himself. He says, "listening is fifty percent of communication." It's true.

Communication is fascinating because we all speak and listen from different places and perspectives within us. For example, when we're in a conversation with someone there can be different lines of communication and understanding. We often listen and speak from different places. Thoughts vs. feelings. Some people don't listen at all. When someone else is speaking, they're anxiously preparing their next line instead of listening. I have outlined a few different lines of communication.

A **head-to-head** or brain to brain conversation is when you speak your mind with someone who listens in the same way. These tend to be more logical, rational conversations. They're matter of fact or information oriented and devoid of much feeling or passion.

A **head to heart** or brain to heart means you may speak matter of factually, but it's affecting the listener viscerally. They feel what you're saying sometimes even more than you do. The converse would be to speak from a feeling place and be received from a head space.

Finally, we can have a **heart-to-heart** conversation. Both of you are communicating from being connected to the body. You feel each other and a greater depth of understanding ensues. This is the most vulnerable, honest, caring way to communicate.

I'm not necessarily suggesting that you speak from the heart in all of your conversations with people. It may not be appropriate at work or during a business transaction, or say, when buying a car. I'm also not suggesting that you speak at a time when you're overwhelmed with emotion or when you get triggered. In fact, this might not be the best time to try and communicate anything.

Rory Kilmartin, a Relationship Researcher explains that when we are close to someone, as in a partnership, we're really in a relationship with one another's nervous system and defense mechanisms. When we get triggered, we react based on how we survived our childhood. It's also a "stressed" response but tailored and honed over many years. When we get triggered by our partner or loved one, we either: shut down and retreat, raise our voice and get confrontational, try to control the situation, or some combination of these. Knowing how you and your partner react when you get triggered is vital information to the relationship. The process of speaking more from the heart and less from reactivity becomes a key in reaching one another and having resolution. This requires being grounded in your body, rather than uprooted from some preset condition of your past.

Not everyone grew up in a safe space with the opportunity to express themselves, especially from the heart. If you were not able to ask for what you needed in childhood, it will most likely show up in your adult life as well. This can manifest as anxiety. In the same regard, if you grew up fighting to be heard by raising your voice, you might react in the same way as an adult when you get triggered.

I'm not suggesting there's anything wrong with how you are in the world. I am saying that most of us were, at least in part, trained by our reactions in situations of perceived survival. When we learn to do our Yoga from the heart, we can surrender our defenses for a time every day. This way we can drop into a safe, controlled space within ourselves. We are in essence returning to some innocence, where we can practice being nonreactive deliberately.

All the practices in this book have given you a roadmap to dwell less in the thinking, worrying, reactive brain and more in the sanctuary of your body and heart. While we cannot force someone to speak from their heart, we can speak and listen from ours. Each time we muster the courage to speak from the heart, we develop self-confidence and security. When we're fully present and paying attention to another person, they feel safe enough to be more vulnerable and speak their truth.

Brene Brown, a best-selling Author and Behavioral Researcher says, "Vulnerability is the birthplace of love, belonging, joy, courage, empathy, and creativity. It is the source of hope, empathy, accountability, and authenticity. If we want greater clarity in our purpose or deeper and more meaningful spiritual lives, vulnerability is the path."

That doesn't necessarily mean we should go out and share our deepest vulnerabilities to everyone we talk to, but it does give us a clear indication of the power of expressing from the heart.

When I facilitate Yoga Retreats, I limit the number of people to create an intimate experience. I choose places that are close to nature, which helps people feel safe and is reflective of their own true nature. Breathing and moving together is powerful. I ask the group to actively listen when someone is sharing. When this person feels the group is giving them their undivided attention, it validates them in a huge way. It becomes a sacred healing environment for everyone, because when we're fully present and purposeful, we are better able to see ourselves in others. We almost always hear something that resonates with us, because we're all basically the same. We might have a different story and developed different strategies for getting by in life, but we're built the same.

There's nothing like a good heartfelt conversation between two or more people. It's refreshing to be heard and felt. This is exactly why therapy is so important and will work ten times better if the therapist is able to get you to speak from being connected to your heart and body. When someone is really listening to us, we feel validated. They see us, feel us, hear what we're saying, and we no longer feel alone. It inspires others to come out of their shell. This is gold.

Marianne Williamson, Author and Healer wrote, "…as we let our own light shine, we unconsciously give other people permission to do the same."

When we shift our attention from our own thoughts and feelings and give our full attention to someone else, something very interesting happens. We alter the polarity of our own nervous system. We shift from a "get" mentality to giving the person our attention. This is how we develop empathy and compassion. When we do, that person no longer feels alone or misunderstood. They feel validated. Compassion has a great power to heal in this way. The biggest gift that we can give anyone is our full attention and presence.

When we develop this level of kindness and love for ourselves and others, we begin to heal old wounds. Compassion sometimes has the connotation of being soft or feminine, but that's not true. Compassion for ourselves shows up by knowing what we want and being able to ask for it. It can be challenging to be honest. Have you ever wondered why people say yes to things when they really want to say no? They often do so out of an obligation, guilt, or a need to please others to feel accepted. Believe it or not having compassion might be saying no to someone as a way of maintaining clear boundaries. Being compassionate for someone can be strong and stabilizing. It can be as simple as holding space for someone or helping them to stay accountable for something they want. Sometimes, compassion has the potential to become a confrontation.

The word confrontation, alone, can be triggering for some people, but it does not have to be, nor should it be, combative. The word *con-front* is another way of saying: together in front of. A confrontation is an opportunity to see ourselves in the mirror of another person or people. The best mirrors are neutral, non-judgmental, clear and straight-forward. Therapists and other mental health professionals should be trained to be neutral, yet clear. A friend or family member that knows you well may not be the best mirror for you. They might unknowingly or unconsciously project their own desires onto you. This is exactly why finding the right space or community plays such a vital role in mental health.

Some yoga studios provide a great resource to our society, because they provide a space for deep connection. In some ways, studios have taken the place of churches that have been on a steady decline in recent years. Some yoga studios and teachers serve our society in a very important way. They provide community and a safe place for you to be yourself no matter what posture you can perform. I am in no way saying that all yoga teachers are created equal, but I am saying that yoga classes have a higher potential to be a healing environment. When you go through an experience of breathing and moving with others in a non-competitive environment, it tends to bring people together.

The moral of the story is to find community, Sangha. These are places where you feel accepted, honored and seen. Avoid being alone for too long in the prison of your own mind. When you move your body and breath, energy moves within you. Give that creative energy the opportunity to flow out and become something with others. To be shared. For new ideas, insights, and thoughts to flow in, you must get energy to flow out by writing, talking to others, making art, dancing and expressing yourself in whatever ways suit you.

Move energy with your personal Yoga practice at home in your own space, daily. Then, at least once per week, visit your local yoga studio for classes, so you can move and breathe and share yourself with others. Step out and ask a friend or neighbor to meet for coffee or tea. Join a hiking or walking group, or a kayaking club. It doesn't have to be a perfect experience. Get out into nature with other people to move and breathe and be your miraculous self!

Chapter 16
Self-discipline, Not Obsession

"Faith is a state of mind that can be conditioned through self-discipline."

Bruce Lee

You have been given the life form of a human being. You already beat the odds of existing at all, on the planet. You are unique. One of a kind. No one has ever been here living upon the earth quite like you and no one ever will again. You are an original. There's no other logical way to look at our existence. You may not like certain things about your life, your body, your situation, but even "not liking" or experiencing pain is only possible because you exist. Like every other living thing on the planet, we arrived in this material world housed in a body. At some point, you will leave the body. In the meantime, you have an opportunity to actualize your life with Yoga. To purposefully explore possibility of breath movement, sensation and form. It's the appropriate response to our reality. It's all up to you though. The truth is whether you decide to act or not, life is already happening. Time moves regardless of what you do. Aging is the undeniable process of nature. Time is the real currency.

We tell ourselves that we don't have time for the things we want to do, but that's complete bullshit. All you really have is time, and you get to dictate how you spend it. If you're looking to make a change and want to cultivate a daily practice you must schedule it into your daily activities, otherwise, nothing will change.

The reason that you brush your teeth every day, hopefully, is that someone originally held you accountable for doing it. Most likely, your mom or dad or someone who loved and cared for you, taught you this ritual. At some point you accepted the responsibility and made it your own, because doing so is an important part of oral hygiene and overall health. Eventually, cleaning your teeth and gums became a routine that you do every day. You have brushed your teeth on your own long enough to know that it makes your mouth feel clean and fresh. If you don't, bacteria and decay will flourish and cause gum disease, cavities, and so on. You have woven the practice of brushing into the very fabric of your life as a necessary daily routine. When you don't do it, you notice it. You feel the accumulation of grit as your teeth get coated with plaque and debris. The same thing happens with our mind and body. Thoughts build up like plaque and our body becomes stiff.

Having the fortitude and discipline to insert something new into one's life can be a tall order, but the choice itself is simple. If you so choose to fully participate in the nature of your humanness, the one thing that you'll need is: self-discipline. The ability to show up and do your Yoga practice when no one is watching or telling you what to do. When you hold yourself accountable in this way, it is the ultimate act of self-love. It means that you do your practice when you don't feel like it or you're too busy or distracted or tired. When you do, shift will happen.

My teacher, Mark Whitwell, tells the story of how his teacher, TKV Desikachar, helped him instill Yoga practice into his life. Desikachar wrote *The Heart of Yoga*, based on Krishnamacharya's work (the father of modern Yoga). Mark asked the Yoga Master, Desikachar, if he would teach him Yoga. Desikachar agreed. At the conclusion of their first session, Desikachar told Mark something to the effect of:

"Practice what I just taught you every day until I see you again. If you don't, don't come back."

Not only did Mark return, but today Mr. Whitwell is one of the foremost Yoga educators in the world. He carries on the lineage and mission of Krishnamacharya and Desikachar, which is to give Yoga to the people and adapt it to each individual.

Desikachar gave Mark a gift that day. He held Mark accountable. He instilled the gift of self-discipline without drama. In the years that followed, a deep loving and profound friendship ensued. From that relationship, Yoga has been transmitted to thousands and thousands of people across the planet. I am one of those people, and now, so are you. You must understand that the relationship between teacher and student is itself Yoga. When there's a trusting connection between two people the transmission of Yoga is not only possible, but direct and efficient.

Most people need a teacher to help them develop the Yoga practice itself. To learn what to do and how to do it while helping them to stay accountable for doing it, at least for a while. In my experience and perhaps the irony of doing a daily practice is that it generates more freedom, not less. The development of self-discipline is a courageous and rewarding act of self-love. As is Yoga practice itself, because all other relationships will be positively charged. With such a level of personal responsibility we can learn and do almost anything.

One of the problems in our current society is that we lack self-discipline. We allow ourselves to be coerced into believing that we need material possessions and shiny gadgets to be happy. The world of marketers and influencers know how to press the buttons of your desires, so you chase and pursue the idea that being content exists outside of yourself.

As an infant, the very first thing that ever made you smile and feel secure was not a thing at all, it was another soul. I certainly hope someone gave you positive attention. It was when your mom or dad or grandmother or sibling or caretaker or dog or another soul looked into your eyes and validated your very existence by seeing you, touching you, or interacting with you in some way. Up until we were four or five years old, that's all we needed. The need to be seen, felt, heard and touched never goes away.

We can and should give ourselves the same kind of attention, love, and validation. And if for some reason, you did not receive enough, it's time now to learn how to give it to yourself. This kind of love allows us to feel safe, in control and gives us the clarity of mind that most people, especially those with an overactive mind, need. Please summon the courage to spend quality time with yourself employing the principles put forth in this book.

In order to learn anything new and embody it, you must have three things in place: 1. education or knowledge, 2. action or study 3. responsibility or accountability. If any one of these is missing, chances are you will not be able to fully integrate it into your life. Developing a daily practice for yourself is like putting spiritual currency in the bank. You want enough in your bank account, so it's there when you need it most. Breathe and move in different positions each day as a celebration of what's been given to you, this life.

Start with 10 minutes per day. No one can honestly say that they don't have 10 minutes per day to breathe and move deliberately. If you really don't have 10 minutes, you need it the most.

Practice filling your toolbox with a variety of tools, so you can pull out what you need in the moment. Train yourself with the various breathing techniques found in Appendix A, so that they're easily accessible and second nature when you have unexpected anxiety or stress pop up. Conscious active breathing can't not work if you do it, so do some every day!

I believe 100% that everyone should learn and practice breathing in direct coordination with moving in different ways. Your body is already equipped with natures gifts. Everything you need is already inside of you in this very moment. Make the commitment to yourself.

Do Your Own Daily Yoga Practice! It's the absolute best thing that you can do for yourself, your relationships and the planet. It is truly the hope for humanity. Please, always remember:

You Are a Miracle!

References

Cleveland Clinic, 12/17/20, Anxiety Disorders, https://my.clevelandclinic.org/health/diseases/9536-anxiety-disorders

Cleveland Clinic, 4/27/21, Stress Management and Emotional Health, Emotional Stress, https://my.clevelandclinic.org/health/treatments/6409-stress-management-and-emotional-health

Dr Ali Binazir, 8/16/11, Are You a Miracle? On the Probability of Your Being Born, https://www.huffpost.com/entry/probability-being-born_b_877853

Mayo Clinic, Mayo Clinic Medical Professional, 10/13/2017, Generalized Anxiety Disorder, https://www.mayoclinic.org/diseases-conditions/generalized-anxiety-disorder/symptoms-causes/syc-20360803,

Managing stress, National Alliance on Mental Illness, https://www.nami.org/Your-Journey/Individuals-with-Mental-Illness/Taking-Care-of-Your-Body/Managing-Stress.

Mayo Clinic, 12/13/22, Post-traumatic Stress Disorder (PTSD), https://www.mayoclinic.org/diseases-conditions/post-traumatic-stress-disorder/symptoms-causes/syc-20355967

Benson, Herbert M.D., Klipper, Miriam Z., *The Relaxation Response*, New York, NY, Quill an Imprint of Harper Collins Publishing, Second Edition 2001

Desikachar, TKV, *Heart of Yoga,* Developing a Personal Practice, Rochester, VT, Inner Traditions International, 1995, Chapt. 6, pp. 17-23, 53-66, 25-52

Van der kolk, Bessel, M.D., The Body Keeps The Score, New York, NY, Penguin Random House, 2014, pp. 21, 265-278

www.ncbi.nlm.nih.gov, National Library of Medicine, The Effect of Diaphragmatic Breathing on Attention, Negative Affect and Stress in Healthy Adults, Sourced 9/21/20, 9/22/20, https://www.ncbi.nlm.nih.gov/pmc/articles/PMC5455070/

Mr. Parajuli Niranjan, Pradhan Balaram, Feb 1, 2022, Immediate Effect of Ujjayi Pranayama on Attention and Anxiety among University Students: A Randomized Controlled Study, Junior Research Fellow, Centre for Integrative Medicine and Research, All India Institute of Medical Sciences, Sri Aurobindo Marg, Ansari Nagar East, New Delhi, India

Brown RP, Gerbarg PL. Sudarshan Kriya Yogic breathing in the treatment of stress, anxiety, and depression. Part II--clinical applications and guidelines. J Altern Complement Med. 2005 Aug;11(4):711-7. doi: 10.1089/acm.2005.11.711. PMID: 16131297.

Grant H. Brenner, MD, FAPA, Jan. 16, 2019, How Yoga and Breathing Help the Brain Unwind, https://www.psychologytoday.com/us/blog/psychiatry-the-people/201901/how-yoga-and-breathing-help-the-brain-unwind

Mayfield Brain and Spine, Staff, Updated 4/2018, Anatomy of Brain, https://mayfieldclinic.com/pe-anatbrain.htm#:~:text=The%20brain

Mayo Clinic Staff, Healthy Lifestyle Nutrition and Healthy Eating, 10/12/22, Water: How much should you drink, https://www.mayoclinic.org/healthy-lifestyle/nutrition-and-healthy-eating/in-depth/water/art-20044256

Online Etymology Dictionary, https://www.etymonline.com/

US Department of Health and Human Services, Eunice Kennedy Shriver National Institute of Child Health and Human Development, updated 10/01/2018, What are parts of the nervous system, https://www.nichd.nih.gov/health/topics/neuro/conditioninfo/parts

Harvard Health Publishing, Harvard Medical School, 7/20/20, Understanding The Stress Response, Chronic activation of this survival mechanism impairs health, https://www.health.harvard.edu/staying-healthy/understanding-the-stress-response

Hoge EA, Bui E, Mete M, Dutton MA, Baker AW, Simon NM. Mindfulness-Based Stress Reduction vs Escitalopram for the Treatment of Adults With Anxiety Disorders: A Randomized Clinical Trial. JAMA Psychiatry. 2023; 80(1): 13–21. doi:10.1001/jamapsychiatry.2022.3679

Boston University. "Yoga May Elevate Brain GABA Levels, Suggesting Possible Treatment For Depression." ScienceDaily. ScienceDaily, 22 May 2007. <www.sciencedaily.com/releases/2007/05/070521145516.htm>

Cleveland Clinic Staff, Heart Rate Variability (HRV) 9/1/21, https://my.clevelandclinic.org/health/symptoms/21773-heart-rate-variability-hrv

Dr. Heather Ashton, 1999, The Ashton Manual, Chapter 1, The Benzodiazepines: What They Do In The Body, https://www.benzoinfo.com/ashtonmanual/chapter1/#ch1

Esther Goldstein, 2021, Integrative Psychotherapy, What is an Inner Child, https://integrativepsych.co/new-blog/what-is-an-inner-child#:~:text=When%20the%20inner%20child%20runs,is%20attempting%20to%20feel%20safe.

Center For Food Safety, 11/13/22, About Genetically Engineered Foods, https://www.centerforfoodsafety.org/issues/311/ge-foods/about-ge-foods

Economic Research Service, USDA, Laura Dotson, 09/14/22, Recent Trends in GE Adoption, http://www.ers.usda.gov/data-products/adoption-of-genetically-engineered-crops-in-the-us/recent-trends-in-ge-adoption.aspx

Center For food Safety, 12/26/22, GE Food and Your Health, https://www.centerforfoodsafety.org/issues/311/ge-foods/ge-food-and-your-health

World Population Review, 3/1/23, Countries That Ban GMOs, https://worldpopulationreview.com/country-rankings/countries-that-ban-gmos

Caleb Hawkins, United States Environmental Protection Agency, April, 19, 2018, Memorandum, Office of Chemical Safety and Pollution Prevention, Glyphosate: Response to Comments, Usage, and Benefits (PC Codes: 103601 103604, 103605, 103607, 103608, 103613, 417300)

US National Library of Medicine National Institutes of Health, 2017, *Risk of Deficiency in Multiple Concurrent Micronutrients in Children and Adults in the United States.* Bird, J. K., Murphy, R. A., Ciappio, E. D., & McBurney, M. I.:

https://www.ncbi.nlm.nih.gov/pmc/articles/PMC5537775/

Staff at the Cleveland Clinic, Probiotics, 03/09/2020, https://my.clevelandclinic.org/health/articles/14598-probiotics

Dutheil S, Ota KT, Wohleb ES, Rasmussen K, Duman RS. High-Fat Diet Induced Anxiety and Anhedonia: Impact on Brain Homeostasis and Inflammation. Neuropsychopharmacology. 2016 Jun;41(7):1874-87. doi: 10.1038/npp.2015.357. Epub 2015 Dec 14. PMID: 26658303; PMCID: PMC4869056.

Kris-Etherton PM, Petersen KS, Hibbeln JR, Hurley D, Kolick V, Peoples S, Rodriguez N, Woodward-Lopez G. Nutrition and behavioral health disorders: depression and anxiety. Nutr Rev. 2021 Feb 11;79(3):247-260. doi: 10.1093/nutrit/nuaa025. PMID: 32447382; PMCID: PMC8453603.

Aucoin M, LaChance L, Naidoo U, Remy D, Shekdar T, Sayar N, Cardozo V, Rawana T, Chan I, Cooley K. Diet and Anxiety: A Scoping Review. Nutrients. 2021 Dec 10;13(12):4418. doi: 10.3390/nu13124418. PMID: 34959972; PMCID: PMC8706568.

Haghighatdoost F, Feizi A, Esmaillzadeh A, Rashidi-Pourfard N, Keshteli AH, Roohafza H, Adibi P. Drinking plain water is associated with decreased risk of depression and anxiety in adults: Results from a large cross-sectional study. World J Psychiatry. 2018

Sep 20;8(3):88-96. doi: 10.5498/wjp.v8.i3.88. PMID: 30254979; PMCID: PMC6147771.

Harvard Health Publishing, Harvard Medical School, Nutritional Strategies to Ease Anxiety, **Uma Naidoo, MD,** 8/28/2019, https://www.health.harvard.edu/blog/nutritional-strategies-to-ease-anxiety-201604139441#

Harvard T.H. Chan School of Public Health, July 2020, The Nutrition Source, Coffee, https://www.hsph.harvard.edu/nutritionsource/food-features/coffee/#:~:text=%5B10%5D,non%2Ddrinkers.%20%5B11%5D

de Cabo R, Mattson MP. Effects of Intermittent Fasting on Health, Aging, and Disease. N Engl J Med. 2019 Dec 26;381(26):2541-2551. doi: 10.1056/NEJMra1905136. Erratum in: N Engl J Med. 2020 Jan 16;382(3):298. Erratum in: N Engl J Med. 2020 Mar 5;382(10):978. PMID: 31881139.

Mahlouji M, Alizadeh Vaghasloo M, Dadmehr M, Rezaeizadeh H, Nazem E, Tajadini H. Sweating as a Preventive Care and Treatment Strategy in Traditional Persian Medicine. Galen Med J. 2020 Dec 25;9:e2003. doi: 10.31661/gmj.v9i0.2003. PMID: 34466623; PMCID: PMC8343902.

Allan R, Malone J, Alexander J, Vorajee S, Ihsan M, Gregson W, Kwiecien S, Mawhinney C. Cold for centuries: a brief history of cryotherapies to improve health, injury and post-exercise recovery. Eur J Appl

Physiol. 2022 May;122(5):1153-1162. doi: 10.1007/s00421-022-04915-5. Epub 2022 Feb 23. PMID: 35195747; PMCID: PMC9012715.

Soeberg, Dr. Susanna, **Winter Swimming: The Nordic Way Towards a Healthier and Happier Life**, London, MacLehose Press, 2019, English Translation by Elizabeth DeNoma, 2022

Dr.Susanna Soeberg, "home and about page", The Soeberg Institute, https://www.soeberginstitute.com/, 2023, The Thermalist Cure

Global Citizen, Christina Nuñez and Leticia Pfeffer, July 21, 2016, 13 Amazing Coming of Age Traditions From Around the World, https://www.globalcitizen.org/en/content/13-amazing-coming-of-age-traditions-from-around-th/

Arlin Cuncic, Very well mind, 11/9/22, What is Active Listening, https://www.verywellmind.com/what-is-active-listening-3024343#:~:text=Active%20listening

Allen KA, Gray DL, Baumeister RF, Leary MR. The Need to Belong: a Deep Dive into the Origins, Implications, and Future of a Foundational Construct. Educ Psychol Rev. 2022;34(2):1133-1156. doi: 10.1007/s10648-021-09633-6. Epub 2021 Aug 31. PMID: 34483627; PMCID: PMC8405711.

Appendix A

Heart of Yoga Principles

These principles can be applied to a brand-new Yoga practice or to any existing Yoga practice to make Yoga powerful, practical, and entirely your own.

- The breath movement is the body movement. They are one.
- The inhale is from above, the exhale from below.
- The breath envelopes the movement. The breath begins just before the movement starts and ends just after the movement stops.
- Bandha is the natural coordination of muscle groups. Generally, implemented with the exhalation.

Yoga is: asana (postures & movement), pranayama (breathwork), dhyana (meditation), and life in a seamless process.

The Seven Sacred Breathwork Techniques

There are many breathwork techniques. I believe these are the most useful and beneficial to practice and understand. They can be done alone or with others.

1. Easy Breath: This is a simple conscious active breathing technique implemented to relax, ground, and initiate: I AM. A great breath to begin a breathing practice.

<u>Purpose:</u> Centering, calming, grounding, relaxing, meditative.

<u>When to use it?</u> Anytime you feel stressed or anxious. It's a nice way to check-in with yourself, anytime you feel ungrounded, overstimulated or need to calm yourself quickly.

<u>Action:</u> Active on all four parts of the breath cycle, each part is a count of four.

<u>Method:</u>
Sit comfortably in an upright position. Not too soft, not too rigid. Close your eyes or fix them on one point. Breathe in through your nose for a count of four, pause for four, breathe out for four, pause for four. Repeat. Breathe slowly until you feel full of air. Do not struggle or strain. Hold the air in for a count of four. Exhale through your mouth, let the air out slowly for a count of four until you are empty. Not forcefully empty, but comfortably empty. Pause the breath out for a few seconds. Repeat. Make all 4 parts of the breath equal in duration.

Note: If you want to create an even more relaxing sensation, extend the exhalation up to the count of seven, making it nearly twice as long as the inhalation. So, it would be inhale (4), pause (4), exhale (7), pause (4). Repeat.

Duration: Set a timer for 5 or 7 minutes and breathe away.

2. <u>Sigh Breath:</u> This is a quick response breath, because it incorporates a vocalization that communicates that everything is okay, and you are safe.

<u>Purpose:</u> Pleasant, feel good, relaxing, stress relief, tells the reptilian brain to relax.

<u>When to use it?</u> In the moment, when stress or anxiety appears unexpectedly, whenever you want to instill a pleasant feeling within, when you need to calm yourself quickly.

<u>Action:</u> Active inhale, pause, vocalize or sigh on the exhale.

<u>Method:</u> Create a double inhale breath through your nose in quick succession, pause the breath 2-4 seconds, exhale a sigh sound out slowly or vocalize the sound ahhhhh.

Duration: As needed. Do 3-5 times in a row.

3. <u>Belly Breathing:</u> This is a directive breath, meaning that you coordinate it proprioceptively with your physical body by sending the breath to where you want it to go. For Belly Breathing, we fill or direct the breath into the lower lobes of the lungs, which feels like filling the belly. Let your belly relax to receive the inhale. Avoid tightening the neck muscles.

Purpose: Meditative, calming, restorative, grounding, de-stress.

When to use it? Anytime you want to check in, access your feelings, your body, connect to your intuition. In preparation for or in meditation.

Action: Active on inhale.

Method: Sit comfortably or lie down on your back, close your eyes. Place your hands gently on your belly near the navel. If it feels more natural, interlace the fingers loosely. The hands help to steer your awareness into the belly area. As you inhale allow the belly to soften outward and accept the inhalation. In other words, the belly will expand out as you breathe in. The main idea here is that you're breathing easy but filling the lower lobes of the lungs first. The lower lobes of the lungs have more blood vessels and therefore oxygen exchange is more efficient. Instead of the chest rising and falling, the belly moves. You can play with pausing for 1-4 seconds, but it should be easy and natural. Remember the exhale is passive, so relax the air out naturally.

Duration: Breathe 10 slow breaths in a row, 3x for 30 breaths. Approx. 5-10 minutes.

4. Ujjayi Pranayama: The Ocean Breath (Refer to Chapter 8). This is among the most powerful breaths that a human being can perform, because it is both strength and receiving. It can be used and practiced all by itself, yet it is "the" breath that should be used for all Hatha Yoga, Vinyasa Yoga etc. It may be one of the most challenging breaths to learn, because it asks you to develop muscles that are not utilized very much in everyday life. It takes desire and coordination to learn, but once you learn it, it will serve you for the rest of your life and is therefore worth the effort.

Purpose: used for all postural yoga, strengthens and conditions breathing muscles, meditative, charges the system with vitality.

When to use: Can be done on its own. During your asana practice.

Action: Active on all 4 parts of breath cycle.

Method:
Step 1. Breathe in through your nose to fill the lungs, pause, open mouth to exhale from the back of throat making a haaaaaaaaa sound. Think of fogging up a window with your breath in the cold. Practice this a few times to activate the muscle of the larynx.
Step 2. Breathe in and out through the nostrils only making the throat sound. You may have to place or press the tongue against the roof of your mouth just behind the upper front teeth. This will help stabilize the back of the tongue, glottis area, so that you can restrict the air flow in and out at the throat.
Step 3. Fill from the top down. Fill chest, upper back, rib cage, then belly. The ribs and chest lift and expand in every direction on the inhalation. The lower abdominals initiate the exhale, emptying out from the bottom up.

* Once you understand how to make the throat sound, skip Step #1 and only breathe through nostrils.

Duration: Breathe Ujjayi 3-5 times, then rest. Repeat 4 times. Work your way up to 10 breaths, 3 times for a total of 30 breaths.

5. <u>Kapalabhati:</u> It means skull shining and is commonly referred to as the Breath of Fire. This breath is all about energy. It's a rapid-fire breath, meaning the breaths are in quick succession. It is heat building and uses friction.

Purpose: Energy building, heat building, purification, stimulating, awakening.

<u>When to use it?</u> When you either need energy or need to move energy quickly. Use it to clear your mind quickly, before a speech or performance. Use it when you need confidence and power.

<u>Action:</u> Active on exhale, passive on inhale.

<u>Method:</u> You can sit, stand or kneel. From the standing position, feet are wider than your hips, knees slightly bent. Place your hands just above your knees and lean slightly forward so that your abdominal muscles are slack. Through flared nostrils if possible. Exhale and empty most of the air from the lungs by engaging your lower abdominals inward toward the spine, then forcefully and rapidly press them in even more to expel the rest of the small amount of air left from inside your lungs. Think of it as someone giving you the Heimlich Maneuver. As soon as you complete the forceful exhalation, relax the abdominals. A small amount of air should naturally and quickly be drawn back in. Do not allow the lungs to fill up all the way, only a small breath back in. Again, quickly squeeze the abdominals in pushing the air back out. Continue in rapid succession. The sound you hear should be coming from the nostrils, especially on the exhale. Create a rhythm. Exhale, exhale, exhale….

Duration: You can begin with doing 10-20 breaths, rest and repeat 2-3 times. Work your way up from there 60-100 breaths, rest and repeat 2-3 times.

6. Nadi Sodhana (Alternate Nostril Breathing): Long revered as a stress relieving breath. Opens sinuses and lowers blood pressure. Alternate Nostril Breathing increases lung capacity and opens Nadis or energy channels throughout the body.

Purpose: Expands lung capacity, purification, energy distribution, stress relief, balances oxygen, nitrogen and other gases involved in breathing.

When to use it? After asana practice. Before or after meditation. You can use when you want to clear out obstructions from sinuses or increase lung capacity. Anytime you want to balance out the system.

Action: both inhale and exhale are active.

Method: Use your thumb and ring finger on one hand only. Using the right hand, block the right nostril only with your thumb. Draw the air in through left nostril until lungs are full, pause, release right nostril and close the left nostril with your ring finger. Exhale air out through right nostril. Pause. Inhale again through that same right nostril until lungs are full, pause. Switch, exhale out left nostril…inhale left, exhale right…from here switch sides after each inhalation…repeat for 5-10 minutes.

Duration: Set a timer for 5-7 minutes and breathe away.

7. <u>Cold Prep Breath</u>: When diver's want to oxygenate the blood and get rid of carbon dioxide from the lungs in order to hold their breath for a long period of time, this is similar to the breath they use. This is also the breath used for cold water therapy and to stimulate the immune system.

Purpose: Stimulating, activating, oxygenating, cold therapy, immune response.

<u>When to use it?</u> Use prior to cold therapy to prepare the body. Use when you feel like you need an immune system boost.

<u>Action:</u> Active inhale, passive exhale.

<u>Method:</u> Breathe in and out through mouth only. Purse lips a bit and fill lungs quickly and completely, then immediately relax on the exhale. You can think of the inhale in two parts, fill belly first, then chest. It's a circular breathing pattern with no pauses. Breathe in deep and relax on exhale, breathe in deep relax on exhale… Get a rhythm going with consecutive breaths strung together.

Duration: Begin with a round of 10, rest. Work your way up to 20 then 30 times. Eventually you can do 3 sets of 30 times.

Most of these breathwork techniques only take a few minutes to implement and feel the positive healing affects. Any of these breathing techniques can be done for as little as 2-10 minutes or long enough to clear the mind and reset the system. When using Ujjayi Pranayama for Asana or posture practice, do 10-20 minutes. Do not force or bully the body when attempting breathwork or postures. Rest when needed.

For video tutorials go to my YouTube channel: @JosephLauricellaYoga

Appendix B

Four Day Detox Supply List:

1. Activated Charcoal Capsules- opt for charcoal made from coconut shells, a few options are: *Activated Charcoal* by Natural Factors (non-GMO), Wild Activated Charcoal Capsules from 100% Organic Coconut Shells
2. *Flor Essence* by Flora: A Gentle Daily Detox For The Whole Body
3. *Psyllium, Pre & Probiotic Fiber* by Organic India: the reason I like this product is because it has pre & probiotics mixed in with finely ground psyllium husk and seeds, and stevia. It's easy to use and tastes great.

Recommended Supplement List

Vitamins, Minerals and Key Nutrients: (always follow the dosage recommended on the product or consult with your doctor.)
1. A great multi-Vitamin Supplement that covers many of the nutrients below is: Organic multi-vitamin derived from natural sources is distributed by Kirkland or Costco.
2. Vitamin B's full spectrum: B2, B5 (Pantothenic Acid) B6, B9 (Folic Acid or Folate), B12
3. Vitamins: A, C, D, E, K, Omega 3's

4.   Minerals: Calcium, Iron, Magnesium, Zinc, Potassium, Selenium,

5.   Fatty Acids and Oils: Omega 3, Omega 9 Fish Oil

6.   Fiber: Psyllium husk (finely ground), Metamucil is one option, but there are many.

7.   Probiotics: There are many on the market. I use Pre and probiotic mixed with psyllium from Organic India.

8.   Micro-green Phytonutrient Rich Powder: I recommend ones that are non-GMO and organically sourced.

<u>Appendix C</u>

<u>Additional Practices For Better Mental Health</u>

1. Clean up your relationships: Figure out what relationships are toxic and negatively impact you and either renegotiate them or remove them altogether.
2. Shower in the evening before bed. It will help wash off your day both literally and energetically.
3. Light a candle as you're getting ready for bed and blow it out just before you get into bed. It's a symbolic gesture of "lights out", go to sleep.
4. Limit social media, news, and other digital forums. No screen time at least 30-60 minutes before bed.
5. Offer random acts of kindness to others. Try to leave each person you encounter feeling better than they were when you first saw or talked to them.
6. Figure out your triggers. Knowing who and what triggers you is great information. Strike a balance between avoiding them and facing them.
7. Write it out! I cannot express the importance of writing your thoughts and feelings out on paper, actual paper, not on a digital device. The act of writing is in itself therapy.
8. Do the "I Love and Appreciate" writing exercise below as needed. Start out with twice per week.
9. Contact someone in your past that would love to hear from you or you them.

10. Get out into nature as much as possible. There's nothing better than feeling and breathing fresh air, seeing and feeling sunshine, and hearing water, wind or birds chirping. You are nature!

<u>Journaling Exercises</u>

Love and Appreciation Exercise To Move Energy:
Begin this journal entry with the words: Dear _your name_, I love or I appreciate… then finish the sentence with things that you love and or appreciate about yourself. You're basically writing a letter to yourself of all the things you like, love and appreciate about you. Get into a flow without stopping. Write as many sentences as possible that you can using this format. Keep writing until you have at least a half to a full page of things. If you get stuck, keep writing I love…. over and over.

Here are some examples: I love your green eyes. I appreciate the way you listen to others. I love when you make time and care for yourself. I really appreciate how attentive you are with your kids. I love that you're using your gifts to help people. I love that you're getting more in touch with your body.

Get creative. Allow yourself to appreciate you. The more you do this exercise the easier it gets. You're doing it as a way of focusing on what's good in your life. This is a powerful journaling exercise that I highly recommend. At first, do it every day for one week. You'll be surprised how well it works to lift your spirits.

<u>Inner Circle Attraction Exercise:</u> On a large sheet of paper or poster board draw a large circle. Write the things that you want to bring into your life inside of the circle and the things that you want to let go of outside of the circle. It can be anything from material things to practices, habits, behaviors, ways of being etc. When you feel that you have a sufficient number of things on the list, use a pair of scissors to cut the circle out and discard or even burn what you don't want. Place the circle someplace where you see it often. Ex. Bathroom mirror or refrigerator.

Resources, Events and Programs

<u>Yoga Retreats</u>

I offer regular Yoga Retreats in healing environments. They give people an authentic experience of Yoga, deep rest, and transformation in just a few days. We teach and practice the foundational principles of Yoga: breath, bandha and postures, which is like a deep cleaning for body, mind, and spirit. People arrive tight, anxious and carrying the weight of the world. They leave a different person: peaceful, mentally clear, emotionally rinsed and inspired to live empowered.

<u>Teacher Trainings</u>

"If you really want to learn something, understand it, and master it, teach it!" Body Wisdom Teacher Trainings are designed to give students a deep understanding of Yoga in The Great Tradition passed on by caring individuals. You will learn anatomy of the human body as well as alignment in all the standard yoga poses while exploring the philosophy of Yoga. We pay particular attention to breath and bandha technique, as it is the foundation for all hatha Yoga.

<u>Online Programs</u>:

Miracle Mind Body Program: A 12-week breakthrough program designed to dismantle stress and anxiety at the source. Educates, activates, and holds you accountable for daily practices integrated right into your daily life.

Body Wisdom Training Program: An online course designed for those who want structure, support, and accountability while you learn and cultivate a Yoga practice into your life. You can choose to take the program solo or with others.

The Self-care Program For Caregivers: This course is for anyone whose job it is to care for others and wants to learn self-care for themselves, body, mind and spirit. For: nurses, doulas, healthcare workers, first responders, massage therapists, healers, or anyone who gives to others.

Workshops and Speaking Engagements: Educational forums and workshops for management teams, schools, non-profit organizations and events about the importance of self-care, breathwork, and movement for anxiety, stress and team building.
Contact me at: joseph@bodywisdomtraining.com

www.josephlauricella.com

About the Author

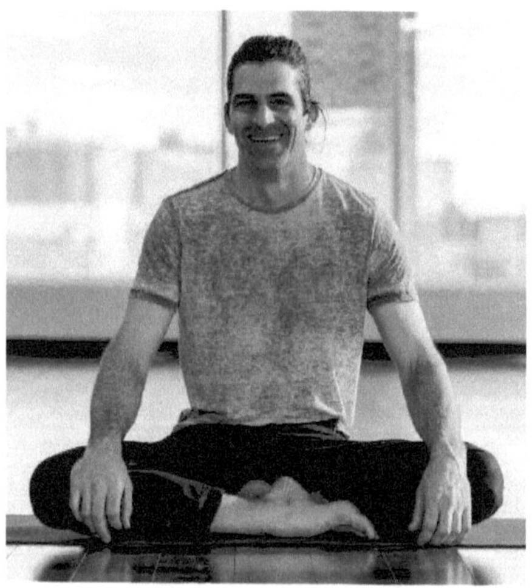

Joseph Lauricella is an author, world class Yoga and Meditation teacher, stress and anxiety relief expert, and wellness speaker. He is known for his ability to connect, intuit, and lead people towards peace, health and happiness. Joseph is becoming an internationally recognized voice when it comes to educating people about the transformational power and accessibility of Yoga, breathwork, and meditation.